Ssh! Lose Weight in 20 Minutes

Alex Buckley

Cover designed by Katie Driscoll

Paperback ISBN 9781908218285

Mobipocket ISBN 9781908218292

ePub ISBN 9781908218308

Published in the UK by MX Publishing

335 Princess Park Manor, Royal Drive,

London, N11 3GX

www.mxpublishing.com

Dedicated to my best friend, soul mate
and beautiful wife Shauna,
not forgetting my gorgeous children,
Jack, Oliver and Nathaniel

~ I did this for all of you ~

Acknowledgements

So many people need to be thanked. In particular, my wife and children who mean absolutely everything to me.

My parents, brother and sister: your unrelenting encouragement for everything I do, along with your advice, support and friendly ears, when I need to rant and rave, are always appreciated.

Steve at *MX Publishing:* your advice about the world of publishing has been second to none.

Sue, Jill and Keith at *The Bookbag*: your amazing editing service has been invaluable.

John: your professional viewpoint and observations not only gave me confidence in what I set out to do, but also enhanced the book. Thank you.

Katie: your cover brings my book to life. Thank you for all your hard work and patience.

Julie: your recommendations when reading the book in its embryonic stage, is really appreciated.

To all my friends, especially Mark, Dave, Steve, Owen and Miles, who have fondly called me Fat Al over the last 20 years. I honestly didn't realise that I **was** fat! Thank you for our precious friendship and the many things I have learnt from each of you.

The experiences I reflect on within this book are thanks to many different people and not just the people I identify above. Without you, this book, or more importantly *Ssh! Lifestyle20*, would not exist.

I simply hope it makes a difference to other people who want to lose weight.

Contents

Chapter I

Introduction

*"Before everything else; getting ready
is the secret of success."*
Henry Ford

This book will give you an easy and coherent way to lose weight and achieve a healthier lifestyle with the least amount of disruption to your everyday life. I will show you how you can change your life in just 20 minutes.

That is honestly all it takes.

The book contains nothing but common sense and because of that, I am convinced you will agree with 99 percent of what you read. So, if most of it is common sense, why have I written the book?

Well, I would like to compare the book, or the idea, to a new invention. Whenever a clever new gadget or device is born into the world, it is often the simplest one that makes the most impact. Then follow the usual retorts of, "Why didn't I think of that?"

The simplest and best inventions are usually staring us in the face, but it often takes someone who can think outside the box to make the rest of us open our eyes and see a solution to the problem.

I decided to sit down and document how I have changed my life, lost weight and become healthier, all in the space of a few short (and enjoyable) months.

This is not a diet; it is a lifestyle, which means you will be able to keep the weight off once you have lost it. I have named this lifestyle *Ssh! Lifestyle20*.

With *Ssh! Lifestyle20* I believe I have stumbled across something that all of us know but very few of us put into practice, because we just don't know where to start. This was certainly the case for me.

So, it was important for me to write it down, because no one had told me how I, Alex Buckley, should or could lose weight.

It's nothing clever, but if I had read this book 15 years ago I would never have become overweight in the first place. This is why I believe my book will help many people in today's fast-moving, non-stop society.

I have found that most people have an opinion about the best way to lose weight. Many people said to me things like, "Go to the gym", "Join Weight Watchers", "Go on the Atkins diet" and "Cut out fatty foods from your intake" et cetera.

None of these has worked for me, mainly because I always found them difficult to introduce into my lifestyle. I like how I lived, what I ate and drank and I didn't want to change. Why should I?

I've tried some of these diets and eating fads and, for me, they always end in the same result: short-term weight loss, only for me to become fat again after the inevitable return to my normal way of life and eating habits.

Qualifications

Am I a qualified doctor, hypnotherapist, psychologist or dietician? No. I put my credentials after my name on the spine of the book to make a point: I am totally unqualified to tell you about nutrition and fitness. I studied music at university!

So, does that qualify me to give advice on such things? Well, I believe it does. I am a normal person and this is my account of what has worked for me and how I have lost more than 42 pounds (19 kilograms or three stone).

When it comes to fitness, I am fundamentally a lazy person (just ask my wife) and, when it comes to health, well, I used to be clinically obese. Now, I have changed my life around and begun a different, healthier and fitter lifestyle. I will share with you the tricks and routines that will enable you to do the same.

This qualifies me, at least, to pass on my experiences and give an alternative view on losing weight, getting fit and how I have overcome the hurdles along the way.

The best aspect of *Ssh! Lifestyle20* is that anyone can achieve weight loss by implementing my recommendations, without any major disruption to their normal everyday eating and drinking routines or the way they like to live their life.

You will achieve success with this method.

I have written the book to be as informative, yet concise, as possible. Therefore, you will read it quickly and, if you are at all like me, start taking advantage of the recommendations right away.

Who Moved My Cheese?

I once read a book by Spencer Johnson called *Who Moved My Cheese?* It is a very positive book with one clear message: accept and embrace change, or fail. People who have read it recommend it because it has a simple message delivered in a short and easy-to-read format. They said, "Have you read it? You should; it's an easy read." So I read it and it was an excellent book.

I wanted to replicate that type of experience in my book and, if you don't want to read it from cover to cover, then I can easily summarise the contents for you: eat less and exercise more. Easy, right? So, why don't more people achieve success by doing that? People need tools to be able to achieve success. Those tools are usually in the form of guidance, advice, tricks and routines. In my experience, people need help with even the easiest activities.

At a basic level, think of a baby learning to eat: an action that anyone would think is the most natural thing in the world. It is something every one of us should be born naturally to do. Well, you can't feed yourself when you are born. You can breathe, be sick and defecate, but that's about it. You have to **learn** to eat!

Another example is learning to ride a bike – an activity we all take for granted once we have achieved the skill set to do it.

Our parents teach us these skills from a very early age, but we need guidance, advice, tricks and routines to achieve them. We need to be taught.

Same Issues, Different Perspective

Ssh! Lifestyle20 will give you a different outlook on the same issues people have always faced when losing weight. This outlook is what will enable you to tackle those issues head-on.

Many of the techniques within this book, on their own, are not unique, and you may well have heard much of the advice before, because it is common sense. What *Ssh! Lifestyle20* does is give you a simple toolkit that will allow you to achieve sustained long-term fitness and weight loss.

If you think about it, many successful businesses are built on the same foundations, ideas, services and business models. What McDonald's does is not very different to Burger King's offering. To take an extreme example and to emphasise this point, look at Shell and BP, or for that matter any other oil company: they even sell the exact same product. They each run successful businesses because they have different outlooks, brandings and price points.

INTRODUCTION

I have learnt how to change my lifestyle to embrace fitness and health, importantly without any radical changes or disruption to how I live. This is why I have been successful and is what I would like to share with you. This book summarises an ordinary person's point of view on how to achieve the seemingly unachievable.

I have selected one key message from each step. This way, when you have finished the book you will have a summary and quick reminder of the contents, so that you can easily recap how to succeed in your quest to lose weight.

Good luck. I hope you enjoy *Ssh! Lifestyle20* and it proves as successful for you as it has been for me. Don't forget, it's only 20 minutes!

Chapter II

Diets – They Don't Work!

"The second day of a diet is always easier than the first.
By the second day you're off it."
Jackie Gleason

I want to look first at the reasons diets just don't work. I also want to look at some famous dietary plans that charge money to sign up to. I will give you my insight into why I think there is just no point in wasting your money by joining these initiatives.

It is important to highlight this, because you have to stop dieting. *Ssh! Lifestyle20* is a lifestyle and not a diet. If you can take on board all the recommendations in the book, you will have no need to diet ever again. Hooray!

The Commercial Diet

Everyone knows that the way to lose weight is to eat healthily and exercise. It's common knowledge. So why do people insist on spending large amounts of money on Weight Watcher programmes, diet regimes and similar commercially-run businesses?

Some of these schemes don't even advocate healthy eating; they give you protein shakes to drink instead of promoting a healthy diet! Just crazy.

These types of diets are just not sustainable and so, fundamentally, do not work. The likelihood is that, in the short term, you will see results and sometimes those results might be impressive. However, most people lapse back to their original weight, very near their starting weight or even over their original weight after finishing the diet.

Totally pointless.

When you go on a diet, you are training your body to accept a different routine; a different intake of food to what you are used to. If you train your body to accept a new routine, it will begin to rely on that dietary intake. Your body will change and adapt itself very quickly to the amount of food, and the ingredients you are eating. This is why you lose weight. Therefore, when you stop the diet and revert back to your normal intake of food, your body will put weight on faster than before, to make up for lost time.

In simple terms, this is why diets do not work.

Atkins

Take the Atkins diet as an example. I have done this diet before and I can tell you, in the short term, it does work very well. The Atkins diet is based on a low carbohydrate intake and a much higher intake of protein and fats than in everyday nutritional consumption.

Basically, you can eat as much meat as you like, but you cut out of your diet carbohydrates such as bread, potatoes and pasta. The body takes time to break down starchy items. So, the theory is, if you stop eating carbohydrates, your body will focus on burning fat instead of carbohydrates, meaning that you lose weight.

This is all well and good, but can or should someone live their whole life on a diet like this? Is it possible to eat like this forever? And, is it really good for you? I would strongly discourage it.

The main problem with the Atkins diet is that when you do start introducing carbohydrates back into your system, your body will naturally say, "Hey! This is something I haven't had for a long time and I need these carbs. I'm going to use every last ounce of them, just in case I get starved again anytime soon – I **love** carbs!" Your body will then automatically turn those carbohydrates directly into fat for storage, just in case. It will also take even longer than before to break them down because your body will not be used to doing it, meaning you gain weight!

It is important for me to highlight that Dr Atkins (the founder of the world-famous and legendary Atkins diet) was one of the biggest promoters of his diet. He believed passionately in his diet. Dr Atkins, when he died, weighed 258 pounds (117 kilograms or 18.4 stone). He was six foot tall, meaning he was officially obese. Yes, he died a fat man. The Atkins diet is, like so many commercial diets, just not sustainable.

Jenny Craig, another giant in the world of commercial dieting, claims to have a diet that is, "Tailored to you!" Well in that case, I would like to eat as many cakes, sweets, chocolates and muffins as I can and, oh, I would still like to lose weight and be thin, please. That would be a diet tailored to me!

If you look at most commercial diets, major food deprivation is a common theme, so once you start reintroducing those foods back into your diet, you are likely to experience weight gain. This flaw seems to be prevalent.

The list of diets and daily calorie intake counting goes on. It will never stop, because people pay good money in the hope that they will lose weight. I just wanted to pinpoint what I see as the fundamental failings of most diets. I am sure that, when you look at what you have done in the past to lose weight, you will agree with my observations.

Once you have read my book, you will see that *Ssh! Lifestyle20* provides you with a plan that will fit seamlessly with your normal food intake. This is how you will achieve and sustain your ideal natural weight.

I Enjoy Unhealthy Food

I advocate healthy eating; it's just that I also advocate unhealthy eating. I enjoy having chocolates after food and an aperitif before dinner, along with a few glasses of wine during a meal. And why not? You should enjoy every mouthful of food and every taste sensation. After all, eating is one of life's greatest pleasures.

This is why I wanted to find a way to allow me to do what I have always done, because I enjoy it, and still lose weight.

Diets, by their very nature, cut out the fattening foodstuffs or just things you like to eat. They miss out on the dishes you love and cut out the snack foods that you enjoy. This gets the body used to something that is ultimately unachievable and not sustainable.

Not with *Ssh! Lifestyle20*.

Chapter III

Step 1 – Time to Change

"You may delay, but time will not."
Benjamin Franklin

In this chapter I want to share with you some of the very personal factors that led me to a point where I said to myself, "Enough is enough, it's time to lose some weight."

Look in the Mirror

Your body is the vehicle that accompanies you on life's journey. Over your lifetime, you grow, learn and act on events that mould you mentally into the person you are.

Physically, your body does the same. Your body is a representation of who you are. It is very important to realise this.

This introduces the first key message of the book:

> 1. *Your body reflects who you are; it's your canvas. Be ready to change.*

Our experiences determine the kind of person we are. This, in turn, determines where we want to go and the kind of person we want to end up being. It is up to us if we are kind, cruel, selfish or even fat.

There are always extremes and for many people obesity and anorexia are serious medical conditions that are difficult to control. I am not suggesting for one minute that they can just stop these major, life-debilitating dietary conditions.

However, for the majority of people, this is not the case and in fact we can control this aspect of our lives. It is simply that we have not been given the right set of tools to manage our weight.

Physically, our bodies reflect who we are. My body is, to an outsider, the canvas of who I am. Even close friends and family associate your physical presence with the emotional inner you.

My family call me Big Al. My friends call me Fat Al. Both are terms of endearment that I like and enjoy hearing. In fact, when I started on this journey of losing weight, I questioned whether I would want to lose those nicknames. The answer: no. It's who I am.

If, by losing weight, I lose those tag lines, it doesn't mean that my personality will have changed. I will simply be thinner, but I will still be the same person. I therefore hope that my friends will still call me Fat Al. I will have simply redefined who I am physically, but not emotionally.

Time Changes Everything

Our physical appearance changes over the years. I am sure my mother and father were very proud when I was growing up that they had to go out and buy me larger and larger trousers. I have three boys myself and I am certain my wife will be very proud of them when they grow taller and bigger than she is. However, my growing has actually never stopped.

During my teenage years, I clearly remember having a waist size of 28 inches. Slowly but surely, as I have grown older, I have had to buy jeans with waist sizes 30, 32, 34 and 36 and so on. Would I want that for my kids? No. Is there an end to this? Yes, thankfully, I have now reversed that trend.

Slowly but surely over time and as I get older, not only have my experiences shaped me, but my physical shape has defined me. I have lived through emotional challenges and changes which are not visible to family, close friends or strangers.

However, my body displays many of these experiences to the outside world: things like scars, scratches, bruises and even birthmarks. Your size and weight also tell a story of how you are as a person.

People immediately make radical assumptions based on your exterior looks, especially when it comes to people's physique. "He's fat," "She's beautiful," or "He's handsome," are all remarks we've heard or even thought ourselves.

Appearance is very important to all of us. You, and only you, have the ability to control the way you look. You don't have the ability to control the aforementioned scars of life, but your size and the way you look are at your discretion.

This is exactly why weight is a key factor in our culture: it is perceived as something that you can control, which is why people can be so cruel if you are overweight.

As I have suggested before, I am not talking about extreme afflictions here, but about people who just carry too much excess fat with them. There are many thousands of us, especially in today's surplus society.

Weight is key in defining you as a person. The physical person I am today can be different tomorrow.
You can change people's view of you. You have to believe this.

It is important that you have come to a point that makes you want to do something about your size.

Are You in Denial?

Subliminally, I have been aware of my weight gain over the last three decades, but I have always denied it to myself, partly because I have always carried it well. I have never looked obese, whilst fully clothed. But I have been obese for the last 10 years.

I would like to share with you some of the other events in my life that, over time, made me realise I wanted to do something about my size and fitness level. I would encourage you to reflect on your life and think about similar experiences.

Back in Time

About 12 years ago, I was travelling with a colleague on business in Finland and we were due to be at a very important, business-changing meeting. We were in a hire car and traffic was bad. My colleague, who was my senior, both in terms of position in the company and age (about 10 years older), made the executive decision that we should ditch the car and make a run for it – about two kilometres.

It was more important to turn up on time and sweaty, than sweat-free and 20 minutes late. So, we got out of the car and made a run (actually a jog) for it. During our jog, I could tell that my colleague was really struggling and I was really surprised because he didn't look overweight or unfit to me.

We made the meeting with five minutes to spare – enough time for me to recover, but he struggled to regain his composure and was obviously totally spent. He was exhausted. I vividly remember this event because I could see myself in him and I did not want to be that unfit or unhealthy when I reached his age.

Little did I know then, that was the path I was already on, and I was to turn out exactly as he was. I was living the same type of lifestyle. I just assumed that I could carry on, change nothing and I would somehow end up different.

That is not how life works.

School Sports Day

My eldest son is six. At his first sports day, two years ago, I went late into work so I could attend the morning's activities. Being our first-born, I had never attended a child's sports day before. It was a sunny day and I was dressed in my suit, shirt, tie and black shoes so I could jump straight on the train and go off to work right after the final race.

My wife and I were in good spirits because the next day we were off to Spain for a two week holiday. Life could not have been better that particular morning.

All the morning's events had finished. Then started a ritual that I have since been told is common practice at these types of gatherings: the mum's race, quickly followed by, you've guessed it, the dad's race.

My wife, having recently given birth to our second son, declined to partake. Very sensible. I, on the other hand, thought it would be fun to join in. So there I was, lined up on the start line with about six other fathers, some of whom had come fully prepared in tracksuits or shorts and t-shirt (obviously not their first sports day!) and I in my suit and inappropriate black work shoes.

"**Go.**" We were off. Now, it's only 100m. A quick sprint. However unfit I was, I knew I could last that long. I was doing very well, second behind one of the fathers dressed in proper sports attire. Then I heard my hamstring go "**snap**" – it just gave up on me.

I had two choices: pull up, or continue as best as I could. I was not going to stop, especially since my son was watching, along with all his school friends, my wife, and all her school mum friends. So, I carried on as best I could.

This was a very competitive race. One father, I remember, dived for the finish line! After I had finished (in second or third – I really can't remember and actually, who cares?) I walked, or more accurately limped in sheer pain, without giving anything away to anyone, over to my wife. I quietly whispered in her ear "I've really hurt myself. My hamstring is a total goner" She smiled quaintly, not realising quite how bad I was.

I struggled on and somehow managed to get out of the playground without too many people realising that I had hurt myself very badly. It was all exceptionally embarrassing, especially when I finally made it into work and told them what I had done and how I had done it. They, of course, found it remarkably amusing.

Suffice it to say, for the first week of our holiday in Spain, I was on crutches. It was not quite the holiday that I had imagined.

These types of events do make you think about the way you live your life. It was a real eye-opener for me. I was forced to realise that my fitness level was exceptionally low.

Judge Yourself Before Others

I am a great people-watcher. I believe most of us are. We love to sit and watch people, making assumptions about the way they live their life based on our observations of them.

In my thoughts, I can be very harsh about people. For example, I might sit on a train and look at someone who is slightly overweight, wearing a horizontal striped shirt that accentuates their true size. I think, "Do they not know what they look like? Wearing that makes them look so fat!" I am actually very unreasonable in many of the assumptions that I make.

However, I have realised over time that I am very often the worst offender of these fashion faux pas.

I do not like spending money on work clothes; I don't see the point. I like to wear shirts and suits for as long as possible, before throwing them out or giving them to charity. I like to get value for money.

Not so long ago, I remember when I put on a shirt that I knew in my heart was too small for me. I could feel its tight cloth around my belly. I still went out of the house with it on.

With hindsight, I was in denial of the fact I had grown too fat to wear the shirt. It was a shirt from Zara (a fashion house definitely for the slimmer frame). I sat on the train into work looking down at the buttons straining on my shirt and my stomach poking out.

If I had looked at myself on the train, I would have thought, "Why have you put that shirt on? You're much too fat to wear a shirt like that – I'd never do that."

I wore the shirt because I wanted to be thin, to feel thin. As it was, it just made me feel awkward and uncomfortable all day. This is another example of an event that has stuck with me and helped me get to a point where I wanted to do something about my weight.

Rely on Your Experiences

It has taken years and years for me to get to the weight that I live with today. It's the weight that I carry around with me every minute of every day, that introduces me to someone new before I even have a chance to say "hello", and that creates people's first impression of me.

I came to the conclusion that I did not want to be a fat old man. Age, I have no control over; one cannot stop time ticking away. I knew I could control my weight, but I had to do it on my own terms.

I want to demonstrate how to do this. However, you must have reached a stage in your life where you are prepared to do something about it.

I have tried to show you the types of events, over time, that made me get to a point where change was the only option and I urge you to look back over your own life and experiences and pick out certain images that make you think, "I wish I could have changed that," "I would have liked to have felt different," and, "I want to change people's perception of me."

Once you reach that point, something will click, and you will say to yourself, "Now is the time."

You have to be honest with yourself. It is too easy to deny how fat you are. Look at yourself in photos from 10 years ago and compare how you looked then with more recent photos. See the changes for yourself. Really see them. Don't deny them with excuses such as, "That is a bad camera angle," – it's not; you are just overweight.

Get to a stage where you can say, "I am fat." Then you will be ready to start *Ssh! Lifestyle20* and you will very quickly make a change for the better.

Life is Fair

The good news is that, although life is generally not very fair, there is one thing that works massively in everyone's favour and is totally fair and reasonable. Although it takes years and years to gain weight, you can lose that weight very quickly.

Using the techniques I highlight in this book, you can and will lose in a month what takes over a year to gain. Most importantly, you can remain at that weight for as long as you wish. It is up to you.

That, to me, is more than fair. Everyone should take advantage of it. Think to yourself: years to gain weight and only a few short months to lose that weight. It is a small sacrifice.

For me, and for most of us, how we look to others is our choice. We all have a choice of what our canvases portray. I simply needed to find and define my own lifestyle that enabled me to paint the picture of who I am, in a way that I could manage.

Everyone needs a lifestyle that will work for them and *Ssh! Lifestyle20*, I hope, contains the secret for you. It worked for me because I had reached a time in my life when I was ready to change my exterior image. Use your life experiences to reach that point too.

Chapter IV

Step 2 – The Secret Lifestyle

"To keep your secret is wisdom;
but to expect others to keep it is folly."
Samuel Johnson

Big Head

We live in a world where everyone wants to show off. People I work with cycle into work from what seems like hundreds of miles away. I am surrounded by people telling me how much exercise they do. Everyone seems to be in training for the marathon, triathlon or some superheroic fitness event.

Whilst they are in training for those amazing feats of endurance, most also seem to be planning their next challenge, such as walking up Kilimanjaro. I do understand that much of the time they are doing this not just for themselves but for very good charitable causes, and this is admirable. However, what it means is that in this day and age, it is very hard to escape from the ubiquity of the super-fit body – the person who knows they look good in a sports bra and tight fitting top or a pair of skin tight cycle shorts, which accentuate not only their very hard muscles but also their ego.

This book is not for those people. They already have fitness routines and diet plans in place that work for them. This book is for people like me: people who value the less energetic aspects of life too much to spend time in a gym, cycling or generally working out.

By the way, I don't blame people for talking openly about how much physical activity they do. In fact, I know I would be exactly the same. They are proud of their lifestyles and they have found something that works for them. They are prepared to spend the time, money and effort achieving it, so why not talk about? I would.

I, on the other hand, have no desire to go to the gym, train for a triathlon or get super-duper fit. I have no desire to completely alter what I eat. I enjoy who I am and I enjoy what I eat, which is one of the main reasons why I became overweight in the first place.

This chapter is important because it will give you a method to manage your new lifestyle in a secret way to make it sustainable. Success is important to most of us. When you achieve success, it is only human nature to want to talk about it with others.

In many ways, I am not that dissimilar to the fitness fanatics who work out regularly. They like to mention their lifestyles because, quite rightly, they are very proud of them. I can totally relate to this.

Success and Failure

Over the years, I have been involved in many different ventures, for one personal motive: the taste of success. I've run my own music and dot com businesses. On numerous occasions, I have invented, built and tried to market what I have believed to be the next worldwide bestselling gadget.

I believed these gadgets would change the world for people who have fun (a pair of bouncy shoes that I branded Kangashoes), work in kitchens (a dishwasher that attached to the hot water tap), and drive cars (a car arm rest, unsurprisingly named C.A.R.).

I have been passionate about each and every one of my ideas and have been convinced that it would be successful. If I didn't believe, I wouldn't have even tried.

I've joined small businesses that have grown into very large corporations. During their growth, and because I joined early on, I have been boastful about how I will reap the rewards of their success, only to ultimately realise that the true monetary success has been awarded to others.

Because of my belief in myself, I have never been shy about telling everyone and anyone who will listen about my latest money-making venture.

Many of my ventures have failed, which has been disheartening, not just for me but also my family. I am certain that my family would not see it like that, but for me, I have failed many more times than I have succeeded.

However, I have not been put off trying, because there is always a lesson in failure and with every failure comes renewed passion for the next challenge.

Failure has never stopped me from entering the next challenge with a fresh and open outlook. Challenges provide a buzz and, for me, that is what makes life enjoyable. Without belief in my own personal long-term success, I am sure I would be miserable.

If Music Be the Food of Love

This inner belief in success started from a very early age. I started to learn the trumpet when I was 11. I enjoyed it very much. I practised hard. Looking back, I know why I was practising so hard: I believed that I would become one of the greatest and most respected trumpeters the world had seen. Wynton Marsalis was my hero and I was convinced I was going to become a talent like him.

Whilst at university, I started a rock band called Hearsay. This wasn't the band from the Popstars TV programme – the forerunner to The X Factor and the other abundant reality TV shows that we see nowadays. It was a pure coincidence that they chose the same name as a band that I had started 10 years earlier at

Kingston-Upon-Thames University. Amusingly, it does allow me to recount the anecdote of how Hearsay made it to number one with the fastest-selling single of all time!

My Hearsay gigged locally in Kingston and had a successful college career with a large student following. People enjoyed our gigs and kept coming back time and time again to watch us. We were unique at that time because we were a 10 piece band. I was the lead singer who also played the keyboards. We had a drummer, bass guitarist, lead guitarist, saxophonist, trumpeter, trombonist and two backing vocalists. It felt to me as if we were going to take over the world of pop. In my eyes, the student circuit was a stepping stone to the charts. There was nothing like us on the music scene; with honesty and hindsight, I now know why.

After studying music at university, I went on to do a postgraduate diploma in music composition for film and television at Thames Valley University. It was a course I enjoyed immensely and I was going to become a respected film composer like John Williams or James Horner.

Neither of these careers turned out how I had envisaged. This tunnel vision approach is what allowed me to take up the challenge in the first place. I could enjoy the workload along the way that would take me to the end goal: success.

Without this inflated image of success, I wouldn't have started any of the journeys in the first place. I throw everything I have at any kind of challenge. I never give up even when the odds are stacked against me.

I am an avid golfer and there is nothing I enjoy more than when I am four holes behind in a competition with five holes to play because that is when I perform at my best. I am sure that if you asked my close friends if I was competitive, the resounding answer would be, "Yes."

Success matters to me, as I am sure it does to many people, which is why failures are always very hurtful.

Failure-Free Zone

I am a success at failure, which is why I had to formulate a plan that allowed me to fail when losing weight, just in case I did not succeed the first time, which I knew from my experiences, was eminently possible.

I truly couldn't afford to fail this time because I have three amazing children and I wanted to be fit and healthy primarily for them. I recognised that my canvas needed changing so I could continue to keep up with three energy-fuelled young boys.

I do not expect sympathy for my failures because I am 100 percent fulfilled and could not ask for any more from life. With the risk of sounding like something out of a Hollywood movie, losing weight, I realised, was a personal battle that I needed to win not only for myself but, more importantly, for my family.

This is why failure was just not an option. The stakes were just too high; I had to succeed.

I now feel eternally grateful for my failures because it is precisely those experiences that have taught me how to succeed in the most important facets of life – weight loss and a more active healthier lifestyle.

With *Ssh! Lifestyle20* I have built a lifestyle that it is impossible to fail at. I wanted to build a lifestyle that could guarantee success, that could guarantee weight loss and healthier living.

"Guarantee" is a powerful word. I needed a powerful formula and because of my many experiences of failure, I realised that a solution was staring me in the face.

I needed to keep what I was doing a secret. That way, if I failed, I could start again with no one realising. It would be my secret lifestyle.

This brings me to the second key message:

> 2. *Keep Ssh! Lifestyle20 secret. This allows for multiple failures and enables us to reach the end-game goal. Treat each failure as a lesson.*

We have all met people like those I have described above: people like me who have so many dreams and have never actually gone on to achieve any of them.

We know of these people because they do precisely what I have described here. They proudly tell others of their dreams and the achievements they want to make in their lives before delivering on them.

I asked myself, "How do I look at these people?" Which begs the questions, "How do I look at myself?" and, "How do people look at me?"

These questions got me thinking. "What do I need to do to allow me to achieve success?" When I've failed in the past, everyone I've told knows of my failure because they can see I didn't achieve what I set out to do, either in part, or in full.

It's so simple: don't tell people what you want to achieve. Don't even tell them what you are planning. Keep it secret. This is a private scheme designed for you alone. If it does not work or you cannot keep *Ssh! Lifestyle20* up, you have no one to answer to. You failed, but only you will know. You can then try again. If you do not keep it secret and fail, then trying again becomes much more challenging.

Can You Keep a Secret?

To be truthful, I did tell my wife, because we share our lives. She sees me every day so it would have been hard not to tell her I was going to start a process of losing weight and generally looking after myself better.

I did not tell her the complete plan of what I was hoping to achieve. I did not tell anyone my own personal end-game. To this day, only I know my end-game.

So, if you are to keep this lifestyle change a complete secret, how do you go about it?

Dealing with your secret can present challenges and, depending on how far you decide to take it, at some point you may have to reveal little snippets of what you are doing.

About three months into my plan, I would get people saying to me, "You're losing weight Alex," and, "You look really good; have you lost weight?" to which I would respond with something along the lines of, "It must be stress; I'm obviously working too hard," "I've had toothache and cannot eat as much as usual," or, "I've actually given up on alcohol for a couple of weeks to give my liver a rest – maybe that's why?"

By this time, I had actually already lost about 21 pounds (nine and a half kilograms or one and a half stone) and don't forget I was only three months in!

This introduces another interesting point. Many people, however close to you, will not actually notice your weight loss, especially if they see you every day. If they do realise, they also might not mention it because they are either concerned for you or jealous. This works very much in your favour and, thankfully, allows you to keep your secret lifestyle exactly that – a secret.

More than likely, people will eventually find out that you are losing weight. At this stage, I did not deny it because otherwise it would become too complicated to manage. You don't want to live a lie or be perceived as a liar.

In my case, my wife could not help telling friends and family that I was indeed losing weight and being more active.

What I found was when people did find out, they wanted to join in and jump on the bandwagon. I got comments such as, "Oh, you should try this running club I know," "We should go to the gym together,", "Let's hook up and go running," "How far do you go?" and, "Are you doing weights? You should tone as well, you know."

This I found quite challenging. I didn't want to share my fitness routine with others. The reason it was working was because I was keeping it to myself and that is vital to remember. Don't share your experiences and talk about it. People like to, because fitness is perceived as a social activity.

However tempting it might sound to work out with someone or go running with a friend, the answer has to be, "No." The whole reason *Ssh! Lifestyle20* will work for you is because it is your own personal lifestyle and you have no one else to answer to. You must remain in control.

Apart from anything else, health, fitness and weight are very private subject matters. They are something that you might not want to share with others. They are very personal aspects of life which should, in theory, be easier to keep secret.

Don't ever forget that you might also fail.

You can still hold on to the fact that no one knows what you actually want to achieve in the long run. If someone questions me now about my routine, I respond with something along the lines of, "Yes, I have my own lifestyle that suits me very well, thank you." This once again puts you in a position of strength and in control of the information you do or do not want to give away.

This leads me on to the next important aspect in helping you achieve long term weight loss success: self-evaluation.

Chapter V

Step 3 – Self-Evaluation

"The first and the best victory is to conquer self."
Plato

The mechanism that allows us to fail and immediately try again gives us the key factor to true success. Self-evaluation goes hand-in-hand with this.

Self-evaluation is probably the hardest aspect of this entire scheme, but the quickest and easiest to fulfil. You can do it within 10 seconds. However, it needs to be realistic for you. Only you truly know your limits, which is why self-evaluation is so important.

Who Knows Me?

No one knows you better than yourself. There is a saying, "Our character is what we do when we think no one is looking." This is so true, which is why, using self-evaluation and respecting its rules, you can achieve your chosen goals.

Let me firstly define a few key phrases that I have already made reference to, and will continue to use throughout the rest of this book. They are essential when discussing self-evaluation.

End-game and micro-goals – what are they?

The end-game is what you want to achieve by starting *Ssh! Lifestyle20*. Do you want to drop two dress sizes, lose two inches from your waist or is it to lose 28 pounds (12.5 kilograms or two stone)? What is your end-game?

Think about this carefully before committing yourself. What did you want to achieve by buying this book? I feel confident that you will already have a clear idea of what you want your end-game to be.

The micro-goals are the steps you need to take to achieve your end-game. These micro-goals are the most important aspect of the weight loss programme, because they are the individual steps you need to take to reach your end-game. By giving yourself small goals on the path to your end-game, you will be more likely to succeed, because you will experience success along the way as you reach and pass each micro-goal.

So, what do I mean by self-evaluation?

Basically it means you set the rules. You monitor yourself, assessing your successes and failures. You are in control and you only need answer to yourself. This is why "Step 1 – Time to Change" becomes so important.

If you have not reached a stage in your life where you truly want to change your canvas, then self-evaluation becomes more challenging, but not impossible.

The Business World

Self-evaluation is a technique that is commonly used in offices around the globe. Managers are tasked with getting individuals under their command to analyse their own competencies and then set their own goals for the next six months. It allows individuals to have their own say in what they should achieve and it is meant to give them a feeling of control and power in the business of which they are a part.

It is a clever technique, because if the individual fails to obtain the results that they themselves have set, it becomes easy for their manager to say things like, "It wasn't me that set the bar here. You believed that you could achieve this – what went wrong? Why have you not reached the target?"

In my opinion, it is a management cop-out. In the office setup, I just don't believe that it is a worthwhile technique. Your manager is there to ensure the goals you set are not ridiculously easy, otherwise you would give yourself a simple six months with no pressure, because you can reach the goals you set yourself in a week.

This is why it is totally pointless. If you were allowed to put down tasks that could be achieved in a week, you would then need to be re-assessed a week later, which leads onto micro-management. This is a management style that is challenged in today's marketplace and well understood to be loathed by employees. This, in turn, is likely to bring a workforce to its knees, or, at best, lead to an unmotivated workforce.

Self-evaluation works when losing weight because the simpler the task and the sooner you achieve it, the better it is. However, you then have to set yourself a new micro-goal immediately, to ensure that you stay on the path to your end-game. The end-game will not move, so you can have as many micro-goals as needed to ensure that you are experiencing ongoing success.

Clearly define in your own mind what the end-game is for you. What is your Nirvana? Pin all your hopes on that goal and visualise how you might feel when you achieve the end-game.

Now I want to outline how to achieve your end-game.

The First Micro-Goal

You need to set yourself an easy first micro-goal – one that you will almost find it impossible to fail at. I liken this to the *Who Wants to Be a Millionaire* game show. You are not meant to fail on the first question.

You've decided to go on the show. You rang the competitor's hotline (probably 100 times). To get selected from the thousands who apply means that you shouldn't go away empty handed. This is why the first few questions are generally very easy.

Losing weight is a similar scenario. You have decided to do something about your weight, you've probably dieted before and now you are reading this book. You deserve not to fail at the first hurdle.

My first micro-goal was to lose just one pound in one week. I achieved this and this gave me the confidence to set myself a new micro-goal: two pounds in the following week. This proved to be too easy, given that I found one pound so easy, so the third time I put the bar a little higher: three pounds in a week.

With these micro-goals being achieved on a weekly basis, it gave me confidence, the feeling of success and, more importantly, real enlightenment that my end-game was achievable.

After the first week, I was happy that *Ssh! Lifestyle20* was working and I was hooked. I was on the path to my end-game, with micro-successes scattered along the way. It was exciting.

Don't Overdo It

You need to set yourself a realistic end-game goal. For me, there was no point in setting myself an end-game that was totally unrealistic, say 63 pounds. One, it would not have been healthy to lose that amount of weight, and two, I could not have ever achieved, or wanted to achieve, such a huge amount of weight loss.

Be realistic about your end-game.

Don't forget that if you reach your end-game and you are still unfulfilled, then there is nothing stopping you resetting the bar and redefining another end-game goal. Just remember, this is why the end-game goal is something that needs to be achievable for you.

This introduces key message three:

> 3. Set micro-goals that are easily achievable.
> This way you will ensure that your path to the
> end-game is accessible and enjoyable.

These goals do not need to be written down, so it should be quick and easy to formulate them in the first place. Your first micro-goal should be something like, "I just want to see if I can lose a couple of pounds." This could even be your end-game. Once you have reached that end-game, congratulate yourself and define another end-game and the micro-goals to ensure your path to the new end-game is again, easily achieved.

The technique which I have labelled self-evaluation is nothing new. There are many sayings that reflect this, such as, "Rome was not built in a day", "Slowly slowly catchee monkey," "It's not the battle, it's the war," and most poignantly for this subject matter, "A journey of a thousand miles begins with a single step." For us, each step should be one step closer to the end-game.

I have tried diets and been to the gym, but neither works in the long term because I do not have the mental fortitude to keep myself committed to the diet or fitness regime. Self-evaluation allows you to control your own journey and guarantee success.

When you start, your first micro-goal will be something easily achievable. You will want to keep it going because it is precisely that: easy.

When you go on to read the Food and Activity Plan chapters, you will see no major concessions are required, which is why I can say, it is easy. *Ssh! Lifestyle20* is so very close to what you are already doing day after day.

Self-evaluation is going to be used throughout the book. Everything relies on this technique, from your food consumption, to being more active and planning.

And don't forget that if you fail, *Ssh! Lifestyle20* means that you can always just start again from the beginning.

Even if you succeed, you may just want to give yourself a different end-game, which could be totally unrelated to weight loss. You might want to change other areas of your life. Define micro-goals and this will enable you to plan your route to whatever end-game you want.

The possibilities are endless.

Chapter VI

Step 4 – Planning

*"A good traveller has no fixed plans,
and is not intent on arriving."*
Lao Tzu

I have given planning a specific chapter because it is central to achieving success. I will make references to planning in both the Activity and Food Plan chapters so that you have a working understanding of how to best design these areas of *Ssh! Lifestyle20*.

This chapter will give you the foundations of why preparation is such an important part of sustained success.

Don't Panic

Before we start, I don't mean exhaustive minute-to-minute planning with lists, schedules and, worst of all, deadlines! All I am concerned about is getting the basics right. If you can get the basics in place, then you will be in the right place to ensure that all aspects of *Ssh! Lifestyle20* proceed without a hitch.

Planning minimises the opportunity to make excuses. Excuses are easy to formulate and easy to act on. We are creating a lifestyle where there is a "no excuses" attitude. The intent here is to leave you in a place where there are no excuses when completing micro-goals. This in turn will leave you on the path to your end-game. Planning is essential in allowing this to happen.

To understand how easy it is to plan for *Ssh! Lifestyle20*, I need you to think for a minute about how planning is already prevalent and essential in every aspect of our lives.

Three simple examples follow:

1. We all buy groceries. We consider what we need, write a list, get in the car or catch a bus to the supermarket, collect the groceries, queue, pay for the groceries, load the car or catch the bus home and put the groceries away in the right place. This is all planning that we take for granted.
2. We go on holiday. We book time off work, consider our budget, go to the travel agent or look online, plan the travel and hotel, book the break. That's just arranging the holiday. Nearer the time, there are packing and all the things that go into ensuring that you get the most from your vacation.
3. Cleaning our homes. Firstly, we make sure we have the right cleaning supplies. When it comes to actually doing the cleaning, there is dusting, vacuuming, washing et cetera. To ensure that everything is done to the right standard, you probably do the same rooms in the same order. Within each room, you also more than likely follow the same routine, so you know that everything is completed to the standard that you desire.

Habitual Living

All these activities require planning, most of which you don't even consider as planning because you have already programmed yourself to habitually manage these fundamental elements of living.

Humans are naturally creatures of habit. We like to know what we are doing so as to feel in control and comfortable in our surroundings. This is why we create routines. It gives us a sense of control in an uncontrollable random world.

I am a commuter. I get the same train every day into work. I get on the same carriage and usually sit in the same seat. These types of routines are common to all of us.

It is great news that we are creatures of habit. You can harness this and make it work massively in your favour when undertaking *Ssh! Lifestyle20*. Once you have started and got yourself into a routine, you will honestly find it easy to continue, as long as you have not made your micro-goals too difficult.

Planning and routine go hand-in-hand. Having a plan allows you to carry out the routine without getting caught up in uncertainty. When you introduce uncertainty, the routine becomes much more difficult to manage.

Habitual living is the essence of life. When you want to achieve something exceptional, then you need exceptional planning. Having the little things planned and arranged means you can concentrate on the fundamental aspects of losing weight and getting fit.

This is nothing new. There is evidence from the professional world that when you get the planning right, you can achieve the most amazing feats.

2003 – What a Year!

One of my passions in life is rugby. One of the most amazing sporting achievements in recent times for England was winning the Rugby World Cup in 2003. This was no fluke. The planning that went into winning the World Cup was phenomenal.

Clive Woodward, the England head coach, left absolutely nothing to chance. He considered everything to the nth degree. The smallest details were managed and taken care of, to ensure that, for the players at least, all they had to do was concentrate on performing on the pitch to the best of their ability.

At the time, Clive Woodward did some unprecedented things that were criticised as being overindulgent, unnecessary and, in some cases, ridiculous. This is well documented in Clive Woodward's autobiography, called *Winning!* To give you an insight, here are a couple of examples of how he planned the team's road to success.

He gave each player a laptop so they could do simple things, like stay in touch via email. Having their own laptop meant no excuses about receiving team news, training sessions and the like.

When the team went on tour, he took their own chef with them, so that their diet was easily maintained (no excuses). It also meant food poisoning was never likely.

He noticed that players performed better when coming out at the beginning of the match than when they came out for the start of the second half. So, he made all the players put new clean shirts on at half-time: when they came out for the second half, they would be in a different place, mentally. He called this, "Second Half Thinking". It worked really well and now most teams follow these procedures.

The players' focus became totally obvious. All they had to do was concentrate on their own individual performance. Every other aspect of their lives was planned for them, so that they had no excuses when it came to a competitive situation.

This is why planning is so utterly important. Key message number four is:

----

4. *Plan every minute detail and adopt a habitual lifestyle, so that you leave yourself with no excuses. Now, concentrate on the goal in hand.*

This is your World Cup. This is likely to be one of your biggest challenges, if not your biggest ever challenge. The better you plan the smallest elements, the more likely you will be to succeed. You won't need excuses.

Shock, Horror!

Using repetition and habit you can train yourself, even under immense pressure. Humans are not generally taught how to prepare for shocking events. When these events occur, we are totally unprepared to deal with them. I'll never forget the first time I witnessed a gang fight. It happened on a train; two groups of youths started at each other with bottles and knives. It came out of the blue and ended as quickly as it started.

I was glued to the spot and my brain could not process what was happening fast enough. I didn't know what to do and so I did nothing.

Over time, I have been exposed to more unexpected and extreme situations. The last time something like this happened, I did consciously act differently to how I would have previously reacted.

My wife and I were out for dinner. It was a very special occasion, so we had gone to a very smart hotel restaurant in London. As we were walking through the lobby of the hotel, a biker wearing a helmet ran in wielding a hammer and shouting, "Get away or you get it." Everyone scattered faster than you could have imagined; my wife and I got separated in the chaos.

I needed to be with my wife at this time, because if anything happened to her, I would never forgive myself. The problem was that the hammer-wielding thief was standing directly between me and my wife, so I had to pass him. I went against the natural fight or flight instinct. This was not because of some childhood dream of being a superhero – far from it; I am a coward, I simply had to be with my wife.

As I ran towards him, he confronted me. "Are you on a death wish?", "No, I just want to get to my wife" was my prompt response, holding my hands above my face in a defensive manner. Luckily, he was concentrating on stealing expensive jewellery from the glass cabinet in the foyer, rather than assaulting an unthreatening, overweight man.

Over time and through my past experiences of shocking events, I have consciously trained myself to react very differently in those pressure situations. I know that in my youth, I would never have run towards him.

To take this to an extreme, people in the army are trained for the worst scenarios. Their everyday lives consist of planning, training and repetition, so that if they are faced with a life or death situation, they do not make a mistake. Their training is there to assist them make the correct decision under pressure.

It is possible to train ourselves, even in extraordinary, dangerous and extreme scenarios, to do something that goes against our natural instinct. It should, therefore, be straightforward to use these techniques (routine, repetition and habit) to our advantage, when dealing with something relatively easy, such as losing weight.

In the following chapters you will learn what planning is required and what routines need to be introduced to allow you to achieve your *Ssh! Lifestyle20* end-game.

Chapter VII

Step 5 – Food Plan

"There is no sincerer love than the love of food."
George Bernard Shaw

We have established that diets don't work. We know that we must have reached a time in our lives when we are ready for change. Keeping *Ssh! Lifestyle20* a secret, will give us the best chance to succeed, and by using self-evaluation and planning, we can manage our route to the end-game, without excuses.

This chapter, in conjunction with the next chapter (Activity Plan) are, as you would expect, the parts of *Ssh! Lifestyle20* that will make the most difference to the speed and amount of your weight loss. Therefore, they are the most significant facets.

We are now getting down to the nitty-gritty of losing weight. My intention in this chapter is not to change the way that you currently eat or enjoy food. In conjunction with the rest of the hints, tricks and routines in this book, you will begin to understand how easy it is to change **the way** you eat without changing **what** you eat. This is very different to a diet and why you will succeed.

It's Easy

All you need to do is cut down on (not cut out) three main food types: fat, carbohydrates and sugar. It is honestly as simple as that.

Here is the theory: if you were to go to a very posh, expensive restaurant, the likelihood is that they would serve haute cuisine, i.e. they do not serve massive portions. The food is beautifully presented on your plate, to make it look as seductive as it can be, but there is just not very much of it. The way the food looks is the most important aspect, as it is in every walk of life.

It is said in salesrooms worldwide that a sale is 90 percent presentation. I totally agree. You only buy from people that you like, so it is important for the salesperson to stack the odds in their favour. They do this by making sure, everything in their control, is presented beautifully. Every aspect of the presentation must look amazing. They dress smartly for meetings. They smile. They are polite to the prospects. They ensure the meeting room is clean, tidy and well presented. They do everything in their power to impress the potential buyer. The best salespeople understand this and abide by it.

Think of models on the catwalk. You rarely get large models and it is well-documented that most models on the catwalks are tiny size 0s. This is because the clothes hang much better on smaller frames and consequently look better. Visualisation of products and presentation is fundamental.

It is the same with food on a plate. Every chef will tell you that presentation is the most important aspect of cooking. The food could taste amazing, but if it looks unattractive, there is no way that anyone will put it in their mouth.

We make up our minds so quickly about everything in life. We know how important first impressions are. Is it no wonder that chefs take so much time to present the food beautifully, for us to savour with our eyes? Eating is such a personal thing that food has to look good for us to want to eat it.

If food overwhelms a plate, it will look unappealing which is why, especially in expensive restaurants, small portions are usually served.

So, if haute cuisine is the preferred style and people are paying a fortune for smaller amounts of food, why do people in those restaurants not go away feeling hungry? They leave feeling full and content, even if their wallets are a little lighter!

It is not because they eat more than usual. On the contrary, they eat a lot less. The reason is simple: they eat more slowly to enjoy every mouthful, because it looks so beautiful. It is also an expensive experience that people want to savour and enjoy.

Eating slowly tricks the stomach into thinking that it has had more food than it actually has, because it takes longer to finish the meal.

Eat slower. It works.

In Training

You also need to train yourself to be content with eating less. I am going to outline some techniques that will help you eat less food, without suffering the consequences.

It is up to you to define what you can give up on completely, what you can cut out of your diet altogether, and what you simply cannot do without.

This is why *Ssh! Lifestyle20* will work: you set the bar and you set your own food goals.

I am a real crisp and regular Coke kind of guy. Dealing with this was the biggest challenge that I faced with my lifestyle change. The things that I enjoy and would eat most days include fizzy sugar-packed drinks like Coca-Cola, crisps, chocolate, peanuts, sweets and alcohol.

I know that these foods are bad for my health and I know that eating them makes me fatter. They also make me happy, which is why I consume them. I like eating these things, I enjoy the flavours, so that's why I do it.

Why should I give them up? This was a question that I really struggled with when I wanted to do something about my weight. This got me thinking and ultimately gave me the outline for the Food Plan.

Is that Bad or Good?

We all have our food weaknesses and I am a very strong believer that nothing is bad for you in small quantities. Every person in the world will eat things knowing that they are bad for them. Some will enjoy it and some will dislike themselves for enjoying it. This is how society has become.

The fact of the matter is that anything is good for you, or, more accurately, not bad for you, in small quantities.

Don't forget that times change. For example, there was a time when smoking was wrongly considered good for you! Adverts on the television raved about the benefits of smoking. Just look at any cigarette package these days and the message cannot be clearer: Smoking Kills! This is a complete U-turn.

When it comes to food, this is also the case. I vividly remember that margarine was all the rage at one point, because it was much healthier for you than butter. Butter was suddenly banished from people's shopping lists across the country. Now, there are fears that margarine can cause cancer in continual large quantities, so butter is actually much better for you, because it is a more natural substance. These reports and ever-changing over-analytical theories make me frustrated and angry.

We all know and understand what is 'bad' and what is 'good' for our health. Ssh! Lifestyle20 doesn't require that you should cut out the 'bad' things altogether, because you are likely to crave them, get unhappy and, therefore, revert to your usual eating habits. Worst of all, those 'bad' foods are probably not even that 'bad' after all, especially in small quantities. The advice about the benefits of eating them is likely to be ever changing, so I recommend ignoring it. You know how 'bad' they are, so just manage your intake and simply cut down on those food types.

My Mum

My mother has to have butter, potatoes and red wine in her life. Her existence would not be the same without those three provisions. She is the classic, "Do you want some toast with your butter?" and, "Is it six o'clock yet? It must be time for a glass of red," type of woman. In fact, I am fairly convinced that she could live on butter, red wine and potatoes, without anything else.

It might not be the healthiest diet, but, by goodness, she would die contented. And that is the point. Why should she cut them out? She shouldn't. I would strongly recommend that she keeps these things in her diet. I would then work out how to manage her intake of these "must-haves".

You have to be in a happy place for *Ssh! Lifestyle20* to work. Cutting out those foods that you love will just make you unhappy. Choose *Ssh! Lifestyle20* and you can keep eating those naughty treats, in moderation.

Leave Food? No Way

You need to learn how to leave food on your plate at the end of a meal. We are taught to finish everything on our plate before we can leave the table. This is one of the habits that most parents do try to instill in their kids from a very young age. No one should ever hold that against any parent.

I do the same with my children. It is a rule that is taught to implant a sense of respect for food and to appreciate how lucky we are to have food so accessible to us. It is important for children to learn this.

My Dad

When I reached an age where my parents trusted my personal judgement of when I had eaten enough, I was allowed to leave some food on my plate. In fact, they encouraged me to leave food, if it was going to make me uncomfortable. My father always says, "Don't ruin what you've had, and so leave what you don't want." The trouble is, the work they had done on me as a child, to ensure that I finished everything on my plate and respected my food, was too strong. Their teachings from my childhood always kicks in.

Because I enjoy my food and I understand how lucky I am to be able to eat, as and when I like, I always want to finish what I have been given, even if it is going to make me feel uncomfortable!

If you are in someone else's company and they are treating you to a meal, by cooking for you or footing the bill, it can also be seen as rude to leave food on your plate. We all ask, or at least think, "Did you not like it?" and, "Was there something wrong with the food?"

This is rooted in our culture and it has to be overcome. I found that I needed to retrain myself, so that I could leave food, eat less and only have what I needed. You have to think to yourself, "Only eat what I need." Not, "want" but "need." This is the key.

Concentrate on when you get to a point in a meal when you have had enough to eat, then stop eating, and leave whatever is remaining. Don't stop eating when you feel full, but when you get to a point where you feel contented.

The likelihood is that you will need to build yourself up to this point and below is a summary of how I achieved this.

At every meal you have from now on, leave a little bit of food on the side of your plate. Start from now, today, your very next meal. It doesn't matter how small the amount of food is that you leave, just make sure that you do leave a small amount. Try to make the food you leave either fat or carbohydrates.

I started leaving food for leaving's sake, to teach myself that it is okay to leave food. It was totally against my instinct and everything that I had learnt in my life, up until that point, so I found it very hard. I used to start by leaving just one chip on the plate. Anyone can leave one chip, right? Next mealtime, I'd leave half a potato and so on. Little steps; micro-goals all the way.

Once you start leaving food on your plate, the humanitarian side of your personality will mean that you start serving yourself smaller portions and preparing smaller portions.

This is where you need to get to. Smaller portions mean less food intake, which, in turn, equates to weight loss. A good trick when eating at home is to serve your food on small plates. Not only will it look more attractive, but it will encourage you to serve yourself less, meaning that you will eat a smaller amount. Try it; it works like a treat.

You have to engage with eating fewer fats and carbohydrates at every meal. There is no point in having a salad for lunch one day and, then doing nothing different for a couple of days, whilst still feeling as if you have achieved something. Setting a micro-goal like that is a complete waste of time and effort.

By the way, if I do have a salad, there would be no reason to leave any of it, because it is a healthy choice and contains no fat or carbohydrate.

The funny thing is that once you are in the routine, you will find very quickly that you do not require as much food, as your body has become used to over years and years of over-eating. I now get fuller more quickly and simply do not require as much as I did.

I also found that leaving food was especially hard when it's free, such as food on a plane, when someone else is paying in a restaurant, or if you go to an 'all you can eat' buffet. These times really put you to the test. In these situations, I get a real sense of pride when I do not go overboard and stuff my face, as I used to do. I can now take smaller portions and leave what I don't need. I can also say no.

It has become a habit.

It is well known that professional sportspeople use psychological techniques to improve their performance under pressure, to give them the best possible chance of success. In training yourself to eat less, you need to exhibit the same qualities as sportspeople. You need to be strong and say, "No," when you want extra chips, bread or another chocolate.

I am now going to show you how to train yourself to manage with less food, and how to deal with hunger in-between mealtimes, without snacking.

Hungry?

In the early days of the Food Plan, you might very well feel hungry. This is because your stomach is expecting the same quantities of food as you have always had. So, you will have to deal with that horrid, painful, uncomfortable hungry feeling.

This is how to do it:

Firstly, have a meal and feed yourself until you just don't want any more. You will now be full. What is the feeling of being full? What does it feel like for you? Analyse every detail of the feeling.

Sit down and concentrate on how your body is reacting to the feeling of being full to bursting. It is actually an uncomfortable feeling.

They say that love and hate are two emotions that are very closely related to each other. The feeling of being hungry and the sensation of being full are also very similar.

You need to hold onto this feeling, because it is going to help you. Think about how fat you feel when full and look at your belly while you do this.

That is your last meal that you will eat for eating's sake.

Childbirth and Weight Loss

Let's put this 'painful' feeling of hunger into some kind of perspective. You need to embrace the feeling of hunger and you can do this.

Women in childbirth talk about embracing the pain. In childbirth, the more pain there is, the more in control a woman has to be to deal with that pain, hence the abundance of pain management techniques and breathing exercises that they are all taught beforehand. Concentrating on breathing allows them to think about an everyday simple activity and take their mind off the pain. Without the use of anaesthetics you cannot expect to eliminate the pain, so they try to embrace it during their childbirth experience. When they feel pain (undoubtedly they will, at some point during the process) women are told to go with it.

I am often very busy at work. On my busiest days, when I am rushing from meeting to meeting, there is often no time to eat. I forget about eating until I get home at night and then realise that I've not had anything to eat. I am sure many people have experienced something similar before. For me, this is a prime example of why hunger has a strong psychological basis. When you feel hungry, go with it but don't let it get to you.

I take long deep breaths, hold for a long count of five and then slowly exhale. This helps massively. Try it.

Pain is different for different people. Tackling pain head-on is the best way to deal with pain. If you can do this, then you will be one step closer to dealing with the 'pain' of hunger.

The feeling of hunger isn't as painful as many experiences in life, like breaking a bone. Having gained a greater understanding of the qualities of hunger and the pain that it conveys, you will be able to convince yourself that it isn't that bad. Don't lose sight of the fact that it is much like feeling bloated from over-eating.

The next time you feel hungry, say to yourself, "This is much like the sensation that I have when I am full." Embrace the feeling. It is not pain that you are feeling, it is just a little discomfort.

Next, visualise the hunger and imagine it is that sensation, that pain, which is eating your fat away.

There is a famous saying: "No pain no gain." That hunger is the animal that is eating away your calories and making you thinner.

This is a good return on a feeling that is like feeling full, isn't as painful as childbirth, and certainly does not last as long.

Am I Full Yet?

I love, adore and cherish the food that I eat. However, from a very early age, I have always eaten quickly. I think this stems from my time at school, when food was a commodity – a fuel that interrupted a day's play. The sooner you finished, the sooner you got outside to play football.

As I got older, I didn't slow down. My appreciation for food increased, but the time that I take to eat has never changed. I noticed that larger-framed people usually eat more quickly than thinner people. I had to change my eating habits.

Eating more slowly and taking smaller portions go hand-in-hand with each other. If you can undertake both techniques, you will lose weight quickly, but still enjoy and savour the food you eat.

To summarise my entire Food Plan, it is basically eat exactly the same foods that you always do. Do not change your diet, but make sure that you eat less of the types of food that add weight: fat, carbohydrate and sugar. Eat these smaller portions more slowly.

That's it.

This is why key message five is:

> 5. *Eat the same meals but eat less fat, carbohydrate and sugar. Don't be afraid to leave food.*

As you have accepted that this is your Time to Change (see chapter III), this is worth repeating: start eating less at every meal from now on. Make today your start point and set yourself your end-game now.

At this point, I want to focus on the planning and practice of eating.

Everyone knows that it is important to eat three meals a day. This works in our favour, because the more regularly that you eat, the less likely you are to encounter the feeling of hunger.

All Common Sense

This brings me onto what you eat. It is basically common sense. We all know what is seen as good for you and what is not. I am no dietician. I am not going to start telling you what you should eat or lay out strict dietary plans for you to follow religiously. This is not what *Ssh! Lifestyle20* is about. All I want to do is give you basic concepts, so you can change the quantity of your everyday intake and consider what you are eating more carefully.

It would be irresponsible if I did not give some practical advice on eating healthily within this chapter. I did a lot of research into this when I began *Ssh! Lifestyle20*, because apart from cutting down on the amount of food I was eating, I also thought it would be good to look into what is recommended as a healthy diet.

I found this really useful diagram from the Food Standard Agency (FSA) website:

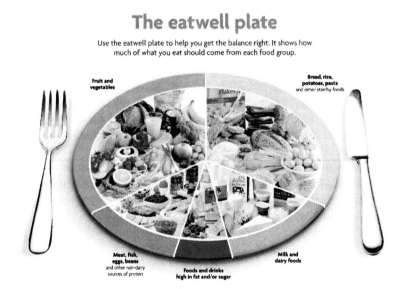

The eatwell plate

Use the eatwell plate to help you get the balance right. It shows how much of what you eat should come from each food group.

It is called the *eatwell plate* and it shows how much of what you eat should come from each food group. This includes everything that you eat during the day, including snacks.

The FSA recommend that the following should form a healthy diet for most people:

- plenty of fruit and vegetables
- plenty of starchy foods such as rice, bread, pasta (try to choose wholegrain varieties when you can) and potatoes
- some protein-rich foods such as meat, fish, eggs and pulses
- some milk and dairy foods
- just a small amount of foods high in fat, salt and sugar

You don't need to get the balance right at every meal, but try to get it right over time, such as a whole day or week. What I like about the chart is that you can see, very quickly, what quantities of different food types you should be having as part of your everyday diet.

It is obvious from the chart that starchy foods and carbohydrates should contribute to your diet. So, it is imperative that you do not cut them out altogether as some diets advocate. Carbohydrates are an essential part of your daily intake. Simply be aware of your intake of them and cut down on them along with fat and sugar.

Apart from cutting down and reducing the amount you eat, you should also try to choose healthy options, which are lower in fat, salt and sugar.

Below are eight tips to eating well, as recommended by the FSA:

1. Base your meals on starchy foods
2. Eat lots of fruit and vegetables
3. Eat more fish
4. Cut down on saturated fat and sugar
5. Eat less salt – no more than 6g a day
6. Get active and try to be a healthy weight
7. Drink plenty of water
8. Don't skip breakfast

Whilst I don't completely agree with point one, it confirms to me that my lifestyle is essentially reflective of those elements that the FSA see as important.

Breakfast like a King

Point eight is especially relevant to me, because I never used to eat breakfast and, to be honest, I still find it very hard to do. In the past, if I did have breakfast it would usually consist of a very large bowl of cereal, or three or four pieces of toast and Marmite (I'm a lover not a hater).

Everyone knows that missing breakfast is bad for you. You have to try and build it into your routine. To do that requires planning. However, it doesn't take a great deal of planning to ensure that you have the right ingredients available at breakfast.

Food Planning

Since beginning my new lifestyle, I will always try to have a bowl of natural yoghurt and honey before I leave for work. This is something that I have really grown to love and, in fact, look forward to in the morning. It has become a habitual part of my life.

It is now vital that I have these ingredients in the house every morning. I have had to add them to what I usually buy. For me, this has been quite a feat, especially when you realise that natural yoghurt does not come in very large cartons, and I get through three to four cartons per week. If we do run out, I just make sure that I pop into the local store on the way home from work. This is really easy and I don't have to rely on my wife or anyone else to remember to purchase them, which could easily form an excuse for me.

I do have backups, which are to buy a yoghurt at my desk when I get into work, and at weekends, if we don't have any in the house, I will just walk to the local shop and get some. Neither is really an issue. I now have a 'no excuses' attitude.

By the way, before *Ssh! Lifestyle20*, the yoghurt at my desk could have easily been a bacon sandwich or, even worse, a McDonald's.

I heard recently that dairy products, such as yoghurt, milk and cheese, can help with weight loss. It has recently been discovered that dairy products soak up the fat in your digestive system, so, you naturally excrete more fat, meaning that you are not absorbing it. By eating dairy foodstuffs, you can lose weight faster. Therefore, I highly recommend yoghurt for breakfast or a glass of milk during lunch.

Having something to eat in the morning does mean that you crave food less during the day and it also means you are less likely to get hungry before lunch.

If you just cannot do without your normal breakfast, then introduce a micro-step and cut down on how much you have. Tips that work for me include tearing the crust off your bacon sandwich, or throwing one slice of the bread away and folding the sandwich so that you cut down the bread (carbohydrate) intake by 50 percent. Even better, pull the fat off the bacon as well. Still order it with your favourite condiments like tomato ketchup or brown sauce, and make sure that you enjoy it over a longer period.

You will soon find that these small steps take you a long way towards your end-game. It comes back to training yourself to leave food by saying, "I really don't need that".

It is very important to experiment with your food, so that you can find alternatives to the less healthy aspects of your diet. We all know that commercial cereals, like Frosties, Sugar Puffs and Crunchy Nut Cornflakes, are packed full of sugar. If you can't cut them out of your diet altogether, then don't. However, do be creative in the way that you eat them. Mix the cereal with healthier alternatives like Grape-Nuts, fruit or yoghurt. Find a way yourself to ensure that you still enjoy your food.

Be Imaginative

So, what about snacking between meals? This is the Achilles' heel of every foodie. The same principles have to apply here: eat the snacks slowly, eat less and substitute, if at all possible, with a healthy alternative.

I used to snack a lot between meals and I still do. I allow myself chocolate and crisps, but I also snack on grapes more often than anything else. I find grapes perfect for snacking, because they are sweet and are shaped like a snack. Each grape is a bite (like a crisp), sweet to taste (always a bonus), easy to pop in the mouth (much like a peanut) and often crunchy (the ultimate snack sensation). They also fill you up, especially if you accompany them with a drink of water.

When I do allow myself to have a really 'bad', enjoyable snack, I will make sure that I cherish every moment, which I didn't before. For that reason, I can honestly say that I enjoy them more now than I ever did in the past.

Take chocolate – and I do! Eat it slowly. Enjoy it. Put a piece on your tongue and push it to the top of your mouth. Let it melt naturally under the warmth of your tongue. Now, take your tongue and push the chocolate around the inside of your cheeks, so that the chocolate coats them. Once the bulk of that chunk has melted, you will have a real clean-up operation inside your mouth for your tongue to sort out. All the time, enjoy the sweet, smooth flavour.

Another technique that I found useful is to take smaller bites of these sinful treats. In the past, I would usually put five or six crisps in my mouth at once. Through my micro-goal system, I cut down until I was just putting one crisp in at a time. It took me longer to eat the packet and I enjoyed it more. Now, I can actually take two or three bites on one crisp.

This works with every type of food. Take two bites of a chocolate chunk, rather than putting it all in your mouth in one go.

These types of eating habits are precisely that: habitual. You will need to practise. It is very easy to forget to eat slowly or take smaller bites. It was so natural for me to eat quickly that I often forgot to slow down, until I had almost finished.

But Do Snacks Work?

To be clear, you **don't** snack because you are hungry.

A chocolate bar, a packet of crisps or a sweet will never fill you up. Snacking is about flavour, about sensation, about the sound of the crunch as you bite, about the sugar rush and about the aroma. Snacking is pleasurable, because of these sensations.

A very close friend of mine enjoys snacking. I would call him a grazer more than a snacker, because he continually snacks. He is not overweight, and never has been. He doesn't only snack on 'bad' treats, he also has healthy treats.

When I go round to his house, especially if he is preparing food, he frequently chomps on raw carrots, cauliflower, beans, cabbage or whatever he might be making at the time. Consequently, when it comes to mealtimes, he never eats much.

This is a prime example of when snacking can work. Make sure that the majority of your snacks are raw vegetables, fruit, nuts or dried fruit.

If you are snacking because you are hungry, then you have to accept that snacking on unhealthy types of food will never fill you up. The more you can convince yourself of this fact, the easier you will find it to cut down on, or even give up, the unhealthy foodstuffs that you enjoy so much.

If you want to treat yourself or are going out for a special occasion and there is going to be big meal, that's fine. Don't worry about it. Simply concentrate on the basics and limit the carbohydrates, fat and sugar.

For example, have a really big steak along with some grilled vegetables and don't have the potatoes. If you have to have potatoes, then reduce how many you have. Follow the principles laid out in this chapter and make sure that you leave some of those three food types on your plate at the end of a meal.

Treat yourself: have a big glass of red wine as well, along with some water, of course. This will not affect your end-game or even micro-goals. After all, a treat like this is what makes life so gratifying. Do not miss out, otherwise you will not sustain *Ssh! Lifestyle20*.

Water

Water is literally a life-saver. It is such a special liquid. I use it a great deal, because you can almost have as much as you like without it affecting your weight. It is practically free and is good for you. I drink it with most meals, because, apart from being refreshing, it helps fill me up. This means I do not have to eat so much.

This is not an amazing new discovery. This is so obvious that it's embarrassing. Everyone knows that water is good for your health, so I am not going to labour the point. It's worth noting, however, how important water is in maintaining the *Ssh! Lifestyle20* Food Plan. Water is sublime, so make the most of it and let it help you achieve your healthier lifestyle. I highly recommend water – go to the top of the food class!

Alcohol

From the sublime to the ridiculous! Alcohol is another favourite and something that I have to mention as part of *Ssh! Lifestyle20*. I love alcohol. For me, it is a social drug. I will often go out after work and drink with colleagues or I'll let my hair down at the weekend.

I don't often drink at home, because my wife doesn't and, for me, drinking alcohol is very much a social activity. Many people do enjoy a drink at home in the evenings. This might consist of half a bottle or a bottle of wine, which is fine and a good way to help one to relax after a long day at work.

Alcohol is very fattening, so as much as you can cut out of your diet the better. I actually did three weeks and three days without a drink when I first started *Ssh! Lifestyle20*. Scarily, thinking about it, it was probably the longest time that I had gone without a drink since the age of 18! If you can cut it out, for a short period at least, you will really see the difference with your weight loss. It will gather pace quickly.

The same principles apply when dealing with alcohol intake as food consumption. Monitor yourself, supplement alcohol with water and train yourself to sip your drinks, focussing on the flavour and the experience, rather than the quantity and the effect.

The Rain in Spain

One of my closest friends moved to the continent about five years ago. There, they never drink beer in pints. They don't understand why the British do this. Before he went, like most of us, he didn't understand why they would drink such small glasses of beer. I went to visit him after he had been there for a couple of years and we, obviously, went to a local bar for a beer. He ordered the small beers and my immediate reaction was, "What are you doing?! We never drink half-pints! What? Why?" I just didn't get it.

He explained his theory: "Alex, if you hadn't noticed, it's really hot here in Spain. If we drink pints of beer, it will get warm. No one likes drinking warm beer. I don't want you drinking warm beer in this heat. Plus, the waiters serve you at your table, so if you finish your half-pint quickly, you don't need to get up or queue at the bar to get a refill. Just call him over and you will have another cold beer in your hand before you know it. It's all very relaxed. Trust me. They have the glasses for it, so let's drink halves tonight."

He was right, of course. The half-pint beer glasses on the continent usually have a stem with which you can hold the glass, to ensure that the beer does not warm unnecessarily in your hand. This tends to make them much more attractive glasses than the UK half-pint glasses, which simply look silly, like a shrunken pint glass.

Somehow, the beer tasted better, even though I was drinking the same brand that I would usually choose in the UK. I wasn't sure if it was because the beer was different or because it was colder and consumed over a longer timeframe. Either way, for the rest of the holiday, I drank small beers. It made total sense.

There is no reason why you shouldn't deploy this trick when you have a drink at home. From now on, when you do your weekly shop, buy small bottles of beer instead of large bottles or cans. This will make you feel as if you are consuming the same amount as usual, but you will drink less. Drink the beers slowly and make sure that you drink no more small bottles than you would have large ones. Surprise, surprise – you might even find that you enjoy the drink more than usual, as I did.

When drinking wine, people often monitor how much of the bottle has been consumed: "I drank half a bottle of wine last night," generally means that you'll finish the remaining half bottle the following evening. Worse still, you might have it in the same evening saying, "Darling, we've already had half. We may as well finish the other half now."

What is the *Ssh! Lifestyle20* solution? Buy boxes of wine instead of bottles. Buying boxes takes the monitoring of how much of a bottle you've had, out of the equation. You will be forced to monitor the number of glasses that you consume. You can easily build your micro-goals around the number of glasses of wine you've drunk, instead of bottles. Set a goal that is, for example, "This week I'll only have two glasses a night." The following week, have one large glass and drink it slowly, along with a glass of water. You can also deploy the same trick, as serving food on smaller plates. Make sure you drink your drinks from small glasses. You will consume less. It works!

Don't Stand Out

The best part of the Food Plan is that you do not need to change anything radical in what you eat or the way you eat. This was very important to me.

When dining with people regularly, as I do for work, I hate the awkwardness at meals if you change what you would normally order or eat. People naturally say, "It's so unlike you to only order a salad. Are you alright?" and, "Why are you not having all three courses?"

With *Ssh! Lifestyle20*, you don't have to deal with any of that. You can order what you would normally order. You can still eat three courses and then just eat a little less. Don't be embarrassed to leave a little at the end.

The Tips

Below, I list some very simple and obvious techniques that helped me cut down on sugar, carbohydrates and fat. Some I have already mentioned, so I include them here as a reminder:

- When you have bread or a sandwich, rip the crust off and then eat the sandwich.
- Take the fat off your bacon before eating it.
- When you are eating at home, serve your food on small plates. This will force you to cut down on your portion size. It works. It is a proven technique.
- Cut out the sugar in tea, coffee and similar drinks.
- Drinking coffee or tea during the day helps control hunger, in much the same way as drinking water. Apart from anything else, it will give you something to consume during the day with flavour and so it helps to prevent snacking. If you are like me and you like to drink a lot of coffee, try switching from milk-drenched drinks like lattes or cappuccinos to Americanos. They are less fattening and just as enjoyable.
- When you are out with friends and everyone is having a drink, allow yourself a couple of your usual drinks (pints for me) and then switch to mixers, which are less fattening.
- Sip drinks.
- Whenever you order an alcoholic drink, also order a glass of water to accompany it. This way, you quench your thirst, dilute the alcohol and fill yourself up more quickly.
- If you have a dedicated pasta meal, like spaghetti bolognese, always finish all the sauce and leave some of the pasta on the plate. If you usually use parmesan cheese, take less cheese (or no cheese) and add salt and pepper as an alternative.

- Have soup for lunch. You will find that you feel less hungry during the afternoon and so, will snack less. It works.
- Snack on grapes, raw carrots, nuts, peanuts, and dried and fresh fruit.
- When you are preparing a meal that involves fresh vegetables, such as carrots, cauliflower and peppers, prepare more of them than you require for the meal. Put the extras in a bowl in the fridge. You now have fresh, healthy snacks whenever you feel peckish.
- Drink water regularly, especially when you are eating, so that you can fill up on it.
- Eat dairy products, as they will contribute to your weight loss. Don't go overboard, but ensure you have them regularly. I eat natural yoghurt and honey for breakfast.
- Drop sugary drinks from your diet, at least in the short term, and substitute them with water. Don't have Ribena, squash or cola. When drinking fizzy drinks, have diet or zero drinks instead.
- Dilute your drinks. You may be surprised to hear that fruit juice is packed with calories and sugar. So, if you drink a lot of fresh fruit juice, dilute it with water. Not only will it last for longer, but you will consume fewer calories.
- If you do have a naughty treat, like chocolate, brush your teeth immediately afterwards. It will stop you from wanting more (and more...)
- Buy your food on the internet, to minimise the risk of running out of your healthy substitutes and snacks.
- Be creative and mix in healthy substitutes with your favourite unhealthy ingredients.

- If you ever buy takeaway food, order the main dishes with no sauces and order vegetable dishes which have sauces. This way, you get to have a healthier sauce with the meal than a meat sauce.
- Observe the eating habits of others, to help give you that mental push to change the way you eat.

I have laid out what I have achieved by using the *Ssh! Lifestyle20* Food Plan. However, you are unique. You know what is achievable for you. Therefore, you need to take this guide as exactly that – a guide.

Build a timetable that you know you can achieve, with easy to implement micro-goals and an achievable end-game.

Monitor yourself and cut down on your everyday intake of food. If you do this, you will achieve incredible results.

Chapter VIII

Step 6 – Activity Plan

"Walking is the best possible exercise.
Habituate yourself to walk very far."
Thomas Jefferson

Everyone knows that burning calories is essential in order to lose weight. The good news is that we burn calories with **everything** that we do. Therefore, it does not take a genius to work out that if you become more active, you will burn more calories, meaning that you will lose more weight.

I don't want you to get concerned that this chapter is going to be full of harsh exercise regimes. It's not. The aim of the Activity Plan is to show you how to introduce more physical activity, with minimal disruption, to your life. This is precisely why *Ssh! Lifestyle20* works and why the Activity Plan is easy to introduce.

This chapter includes a way to not only give you the processes to complete and maintain an activity plan, but also a scheme that will allow you to enjoy and continue to be more active over an extended timeframe.

The Activity Plan is arranged in two stages and by completing both stages it will enable you to lose weight quickly and, vitally, keep that weight off!

Both stages work seamlessly together. Stage 1 is straightforward to introduce and involves more of a psychological shift, rather than physical exertion, while Stage 2 requires a little dedicated physical commitment.

I can assure you that, whoever you are and whatever lifestyle you currently lead, the Activity Plan will provide you with the tools you need to be more active, and this in turn will help you to lose weight.

It is really easy and it is sustainable.

Who's Fat?

Think of children. They don't get fat (or shouldn't get fat) because they are continually running around and burning energy. Adults in our modern society don't generally do that, unless they are professional sportspeople, and there aren't many fat footballers around. You don't see fat wild animals. Why? They run, hunt and are very active. In the past, we were also out hunting for food, meaning we were constantly active. I can bet you that Neanderthal man was not fat.

It is not because of a lack of sport and exercise why the nation has become fatter; there are more adults exercising now than 60 years ago, but there are also more people that are inactive than 60 years ago!

Today, there is a culture of sitting. At work, people sit at desks. We relax by sitting and watching TV or sitting at a computer. People have more access to cars, buses and trains than ever before.

With the constant need to save time and energy, power tools have been invented (hedge trimmers, dish washers, hoovers, cake mixers, mowers) to take the strain out of household tasks. Even email means we don't have to walk to the post box as often as we used to!

In our bid to be more productive, the small bursts of energy that an adult of 60 years ago burnt, in today's society are not being burnt throughout the day and this is where the calorie count really accumulates.

Therefore, if you can get into the habit of regular short bursts of extra activity, you will reap the rewards.

It is what humans are naturally meant to do.

Be More Active: Stage 1

Stage 1 of the Activity Plan is simply about adding more activity into your daily routine and there are many opportunities to do this. Modern society and human biology make it more natural for us to choose the least active option. So, rebel against your natural biological instinct.

When you are next at the supermarket, park your car as far away from the store entrance as possible. How much time will you lose by doing this? Not much. Plus, you are likely to be parked in a space where it is less crowded and easier to park, meaning it will also be less likely for someone to bump or scratch your car. A win-win situation.

Holidays are designed to give us time to relax away from the hurly burly of normality. It seems crazy, then, when we get to the airport at the start of the holiday to get stressed, joining queues and generally increasing blood pressure.

I heard a sport & exercise psychologist on the radio the other day say that even five minutes of gentle activity can raise the mood for two to three hours and lower blood pressure for up to six hours. Therefore, when you are travelling, do not take the escalator or travelator, simply walk instead. It is scientifically proven to make you feel better. You will be in a better mood for the start of your holiday and more relaxed! Another win-win scenario.

After all, it is well known that the one thing that we need to do before and after flying is to have good circulation and what is the best way to help circulation? Walking!

If you walk more and take the stairs, not only will you physically feel better about yourself, but watching those 'lazy' people waiting for the lift, or struggling to get on to the overcrowded escalator, will be a mental boost as well. Besides, it is likely that you will also reach the destination before them!

It is amazing how much time we spend standing around waiting for modern transport devices, time you could spend walking and being more active.

How often do people stand at bus stops knowing their next bus is not due to arrive for another 10 minutes and yet the next stop on the bus route is less than a five minute walk away? The solution in the Activity Plan would be to walk five minutes to the next stop and still catch the same bus. Imagine how much fitter you will be if you take advantage of all these five-minute opportunities throughout the day.

If you already walk, on your way to work, take a more scenic route from the station to office. Don't pick up your takeaway coffee at the station, find an alternative cafe that requires you to walk an extra five minutes. Be creative. You know your lifestyle better than anyone. How can you be more active and personalise Stage 1 of the Activity Plan so that you can sustain it?

As an example, a friend of mine lives half a mile from the train station. That is a 10 minute walk. However, he drives each morning. He is denying himself the opportunity to burn 35 calories each way. That's 350 calories per working week and over a working year (45 weeks), it is 15,750 calories. With 3,500 calories per pound, that is equal to four and a half pounds (two kilograms or a third of a stone) that he is essentially gaining, by not walking, every year of his working life! It really is that simple.

I had to think outside the box to allow myself to be more active on a daily basis. I am not a smoker, but I now take cigarette breaks with my colleagues. I encourage them not to huddle outside the front door of the office, but to walk with me around the block. Consequently, I am adding a little more activity into my day, without any major disruption. It is also fairer, because as a non-smoker you don't generally take regular five minute intervals away from your desk. I do now and I choose not to smoke, but to burn calories.

In the 1950s, there was no choice but to be more active. The baby-boomers and the space age changed this by designing a world of automation, which has given us all the choice to opt out of activity.

You can still enjoy technology and the sedentary lifestyle that it gives us, but make sure you also increase your daily activity. This is the same as the theory of the Food Plan chapter. No radical changes to your life are required. Stage 1 of the Activity Plan is to simply introduce a little more physical activity into your life. five minutes' extra activity each day, without changing anything else, will add up to enough calories in a year to burn off three or four pounds of fat.

How Many Calories?

For interest, I have included a selection of activities in the next table which will give you a rough idea of how many calories you will burn, by getting more active.

20 Minutes of Activity	Kcals Used
Ironing	30
Cleaning Windows	56
Playing Pool	66
Walking	70
Dancing	90
Gardening	106
Cycling	124
Jogging	130
Football	140
Tennis	144
Swimming	150
Running	194
Squash	204

It is important to note that the amount of energy people use can vary widely even if they seem to be a similar build or age. Therefore, the table is a guide only.

Excuses, Excuses

The biggest excuse people have for saying they cannot do activity or exercise is that they do not have enough time. This is because people think exercise has to be done all at once. Calories burned are calories burned, whether you burn them in one go or in bite-size chunks. I recommend that you spend more time being conscious of those more active opportunities, rather than making excuses about not having enough time. Everyone has time. No more excuses.

You need to get out of the habit of taking the lazy option, like the escalator or lift. Once you have achieved this, you will find it amazing how inactive you have been, without even realising.

After you have introduced and made a habit of those five-minute opportunities, you will find that you can recognise them more easily and many more five-minute slots will magically appear in your day. Take advantage of them, because there will be no major impact on your lifestyle.

This is what *Ssh! Lifestyle20* is all about. No matter how small or insignificant you think each extra five-minute slot is, they will make a massive difference to your weight loss.

Stage 1 and 2 of the Activity Plan work in conjunction with each other. After you have trained yourself to be more active on a regular basis, as defined in Stage 1, it is time to introduce Stage 2: a dedicated, 20-minute end-game.

Be More Active: Stage 2

Introducing more activity to your daily life is the first step and the minimum requirement of the Activity Plan. Any physical activity you can add to your current lifestyle will help.

By introducing a completely new activity into your life, you will find it easier to make it a habit. It will be more effective than building a plan that solely relies on extra activities, based around your already hectic, and more than likely, unpredictable lifestyle. It will also help you lose weight faster.

The 20-Minute Rule

You need to aim to introduce a dedicated, more intense activity for 20 minutes every other day. This is all that is required to complete Stage 2. Have a two-week schedule, so that all you will ever do is 80 minutes in week one and 60 minutes in week two. You should not aim to do any more than that per fortnight, ever.

20 minutes every other day.

We can easily train ourselves to accept that 20 minutes is such a little commitment, so it becomes too difficult to avoid it.

I decided to set myself a strict 20-minute schedule of running every other day. This is my end-game. It really does not matter how you construct your Activity Plan, as long as you are doing more than you do now **and** you formulate a plan that you can sustain. Whether it's fitting more activity into your current lifestyle (Stage 1), a dedicated activity (Stage 2), or ideally both, it has to be sustainable.

Being more active has to become part of your life. It will enable you to lose weight quickly and give your body a new lease of life. It is essential. You have to accept this.

When?

I do my 20 minutes when I get home from work in the evenings. I don't want to do them in the morning, because that time is spent with my children. I don't want to do them at lunchtime, because that time is spent socialising with my colleagues from work, and I enjoy my food too much to disrupt that time. With the added complications of taking running gear into work, then changing out of and into my suit before and after a workout, let alone showering, it all becomes too much like a chore. The 20-minute routine soon takes all of my lunch hour. This defeats the purpose of 20 minutes being easy to fit in to your day.

Find a time when you know that you can put 20 minutes aside without it encroaching on your personal time. It might be just before your bedtime routine at 10pm, when you would usually sit and watch the news that you read in a newspaper earlier that day, when it is dark and quiet outside. This is actually a very enjoyable time to take in some 'you' time, out running.

I will mention the 20-minute concept a lot because it is at the core of *Ssh! Lifestyle20*. Psychologically, 20 minutes doesn't feel like a lot of time, and, it's not.

Often, I come home from work and cannot be bothered to go out for 20 minutes of physical activity. It is absurd how hard I find it sometimes to motivate myself to be active.

Because of this, I had to give myself a mechanism that would allow me to overcome this mental defiance. Every sinew in my body would be saying, "I don't want to go out and do the active plan today," but telling myself, "It's only 20 minutes," over and over again helped massively in achieving, and sustaining, the micro-goal.

This brings me onto key message six. It is the most important message of the book, which gives me the opportunity to repeat:

----
6. Be more active – it's only 20 minutes!

Say to yourself, "It's only 20 minutes. That is easy to do."

How Long?

Who can afford 20 minutes? Everyone.

To put this into perspective, 20 minutes every other day is just 140 minutes every two weeks, which is only four hours and 40 minutes a month, or about two and a half days a year. This is approximately the same time (in one year) that you spend getting dressed or according to a recent survey of over 2,000 consumers (by Hostway), the average online shopper spends two and a half days each year waiting for webpages to load! To put it simply, it is really not a lot of time to dedicate to your health.

To encourage you, think of everyday events that you enjoy that also take roughly 20 minutes. I can spend 20 minutes surfing TV channels to find something I might want to watch. I can take 20 minutes reading a menu in a restaurant and deciding what I want to eat. I take 20 minutes getting ready to go out for an evening or researching on the web which film I might want to see in the cinema at the weekend.

The list is endless and it all contributes to one inescapable fact: 20 minutes is not a long time, especially as all you need to do is 20 minutes every other day. This actually means that the entire commitment is only 10 minutes per day.

The only way I could get myself to commit to Stage 2 of the Activity Plan was to make the concept of it so minuscule that I would have no excuse to put it off.

I repeat over and over, "It's only 20 minutes – that's all." By telling yourself that it is only 20 minutes of your life and by realising the enormity of what those 20 minutes can achieve, you will commit to doing it much more readily. In turn, that will help you make it a habit – a routine of life.

As already stated, 20 minutes should be your end-game. To reach that point, you will, more than likely, need to build up to it. I did. When I started, there was no way that I could walk for 20 minutes without getting tired, let alone run! I was completely unfit and could not even run for a bus without getting completely out of breath.

What made me decide that I needed to do something about my weight and fitness was that I ran for a train and, after catching it, I could not believe how exhausted I was and how much a short burst of running had taken out of me. It was an eye-opener for me.

Getting Started

I would like to explain how I achieved the Activity Plan end-game and, as always, share some helpful hints, tricks and advice that helped me along the way.

You should, then, be able to build your own plan and work at it to achieve your personal fitness end-game, which will lead to weight loss.

To get started, all you need to do is take a very small step. I set myself a micro-goal of five minutes' running every other day for the first two weeks. The most important aspect of this first goal was to get me into the routine of getting dressed into the running gear and getting out of the house after I got home from work, whatever the weather!

Five minutes should not be a difficult commitment for anyone, which is why I set the bar low for my first micro-goal. It is the only reason why I completed it. I succeeded and passed the first step. I was incredibly satisfied with myself. Apart from anything else, having five minutes as my first goal also got me used to getting into the routine of running every other day. This was very important.

I then set my micro-goal framework to enable me to reach the golden 20 minute mark. This is how I achieved it:

Week 1 – 5 minute jog, every other day
Week 2 – 5 minute jog, every other day

Week 3 – 10 minute jog, every other day
Week 4 – 10 minute jog, every other day

Week 5 – 15 minute jog, every other day
Week 6 – 15 minute jog, every other day

Week 7 – 20 minute jog, every other day
Week 8 – 20 minute jog, every other day

Don't forget: it is important to allow the body and muscles time to rest so, if your dedicated activity is strenuous, have a rest day in-between.

If you find that running is too hard, then do the same routine as above, but walk instead of run. Build up your strength with brisk walking. No strolling, please. Push yourself, so that you can run as soon as possible. When you are taking regular 20-minute brisk walks and are confident enough, try to run for five minutes instead of walking for 20. Again, slowly build yourself up over time, so, ultimately, you will be able to jog for 20 minutes.

Keeping *Ssh! Lifestyle20* secret helped me tremendously when I started Stage 2 of the Activity

Plan. I found running for only five minutes somewhat embarrassing, but nonetheless it was something of which I, quite rightly, felt very proud.

Ssh! Lifestyle20 allows you to focus on the small steps, without the danger of others passing judgement. They do not know what your end-game is and they have no idea of what you are trying to achieve. I could achieve the micro-goals and be very proud of reaching and passing my milestones. I was edging closer and closer to my personal end-game without anyone knowing.

The Power of Music

Music is a very important part of the Activity Plan. It evokes such powerful emotions, so use it as a tool to help you achieve the 20-minute end-game goal. As you run, you should listen to music that means something to you.

Hearing is a very powerful sense and we all know it can spark vivid memories. I found that anything that helped me get over the initial discomfort of jogging was well-worth implementing. Listening to music, whilst being active, is a wonderful catalyst for forgetting about what you are actually doing and concentrating on something different.

I would also strongly recommend that you listen to the same album every time you do your dedicated activity. The theory behind this is the same as in other areas of *Ssh! Lifestyle20*. You have to start reprogramming your brain and, for the Activity Plan, this means training yourself to accept and like being active. This is the case for Stages 1 and 2 alike.

If you choose an album that means something to you, you will have strong memories associated with it. These memories will be hard to forget, which is why the music recaptures them. If you start exercising and always listen to the same tracks, that will take you to a happy place. If you habitually do this, you will find Stage 2 of the Activity Plan becomes easier to achieve.

In fact, I found one of the hardest aspects of my dedicated activity was getting out of the door in the first place. Having music playing even as I did this simple act put me in a better frame of mind. I found it a very powerful motivator.

It is fascinating how powerful the brain is and that it can bring back such clear memories simply by listening to music. The brain will not allow you to forget these associations easily, so you can use this to your advantage. However many times you listen to that music, you will not be able to stop yourself from connecting to those happy times. This will make it easier for you to achieve your micro-goals in Stage 2 of the Activity Plan.

The better you know the tracks, the quicker the 20 minutes will pass by. You know instinctively how long a song lasts, so, if you allow yourself to immerse your thoughts in the music, you can gauge how much longer you need to be active for. This means you don't need a clock, which is distracting and a surefire way to make it feel like it's taking longer. You end up constantly checking the time to see how long you have taken and how much longer there is to go – it's very disruptive.

The Stranger

I want to give you some specifics of how I used music to help me make my active routine habitual.

The album I run to is Billy Joel's *The Stranger*. It is quite good for timing, because the first four tracks add up to about 21 minutes, meaning I know exactly how long I need to run for, without having to bring a watch.

To put Stage 2 of my active plan into perspective, the first time I jogged I could only run for the length of the first song on the album (*Movin' Out*), which is only 3:30! I can now comfortably run for the first four songs. This is where you need to get to.

To have an album where the first four songs add up to 20 minutes also puts me in a positive place, mentally. The first song is only 3:30, so after that has finished, I feel as if I am 25 percent through the run, because one of the four songs has completed. In reality, I've still got 16:30 to run.

Don't think that you need to run to upbeat, fast music like the music that is blasted out in gyms. You need music that means something to you. *The Stranger* works well for me because there is a mixture of slow and fast music within the first four songs. Coincidentally, by the time I get to the ¾ mark (about 15 minutes in), the album is in an upbeat mode, meaning it helps me get to the finish line.

Choose your album and music carefully. You might not get it right the first time. Experiment, but once you find an album that works for you, stick with it. Make it a habitual part of your active plan.

Another reason to use the same album is that you can reinforce the association of enjoyment by listening to it when you are relaxing at home. Put your feet up and listen to the music. Not only will you enjoy the music, but it also gives you a wonderful sense of how quickly 20 minutes can pass when you are not burning calories at the same time. It strengthens the message that 20 minutes every other day is not a big commitment.

Lifetime Gym Goer?

Once you are regularly running for 20 minutes and your level of fitness has increased sufficiently, you might want to push yourself.

Remember, *Ssh! Lifestyle20* is **not** about that.

Do you really think that a person who has a gym membership is going to be a member for life? And I mean forever. Will they habitually go three, four or five times a week for the rest of their lives? There might be a minority that do, but generally, no, I simply don't believe they will or do. For the gym goers that do go regularly and continue their membership for life, this book is not for them. They have already made fitness a habitual part of their lives and I commend them for that.

The gym is, for most of us, a fad or a social activity. Don't get me wrong – many people might end up going for six months, a year or even more. However, it takes time, money and commitment to continue going to a gym, long term. I know, because I've done it. I also know, because I see people join gyms all the time, only to pay their monthly fees and not use the facilities.

The idea behind *Ssh! Lifestyle20* is that you can continue with it. The entire programme is set up to allow you to fail, so that if you do, all you need to do is reassess your micro-goals and put a different set in place. You can continue eating healthily and being more active regularly, however little it might seem to the outside world.

You can, and should, do this continually, especially Stage 1. There are no excuses for not walking a little more!

Pushing Yourself

I found that I wanted to push myself to see how far I could go. I was captivated by how my body was changing and I wanted to test myself.

I was away on work in Glasgow when I pushed myself. As part of the hotel complex where I was staying, there was a gym, so I decided to try out a running machine.

I had been to gyms before and, to be honest, they make me feel very self-conscious. I can't help but think that people are looking at me and making judgement calls about me, my life and my fitness. This is why I would have never gone in the early days of *Ssh! Lifestyle20*. Imagine feeling self-conscious, then getting on a running machine, only walking for five minutes, then changing and leaving! I couldn't have done it.

If you feel that the gym is right for you, then I would not stop you from using them. However, it seems to go against every aspect of *Ssh! Lifestyle20*. It also seems like such a waste of time getting to the gym, changing, doing your workout, showering, changing and going home again, when 20 minutes is all that is required.

The time that you spend before and after the workout means the total time away from doing other more enjoyable things in your life is increased threefold. There is a lot of rigmarole associated with working out at a gym. I do understand that for many there could be an enjoyable social aspect of going to gyms, but for me, you simply waste too much time faffing around and not actually working out.

I have not even mentioned the costs involved with gym membership, but the whole ethos is contrary to *Ssh! Lifestyle20*.

Many people join gyms because they want to do something about their weight and/or fitness. They join believing that if they start paying a not insignificant amount of money on a monthly basis to a third party, it will somehow make them use the facilities regularly to work out. The intention is right, but, in practice, you still need to have the commitment. This is why so many gym memberships lapse after the first 12 months.

However, on this occasion, I did go to this gym, because:

- I wanted to test myself.
- I was away for work and had nothing better to do. With time on my hands, exercising was not going to be detrimental to my lifestyle. In other words, I had nothing more enjoyable to do with my time alone in Glasgow.
- I did not have to pay for the privilege of using the facilities, as they were part of the hotel.

On entering the gym, I realised how much *Ssh! Lifestyle20* goes against everything that a gym is. People were all working out in very close proximity to each other. Fitness fanatics were all over the place, lifting enormously heavy weights and grunting loudly to ensure that people take a cursory glance. I am probably being very unfair, but that is what it felt like to me.

Treadmill!

I jumped enthusiastically onto the treadmill. I had soon jogged my way to 20 minutes – my normal time. My head was telling me to continue. I felt strong and positive, so I did. 30 minutes came and went and at this point I was saying to myself, "Just get to 40 minutes and then stop." I didn't stop at 40 minutes, because now I had the hour mark in my sights. As I reached the hour, I looked down at my distance and the machine was shouting nine kilometres! Now all I was interested in was completing 10 kilometres, which I did in one hour and six minutes. "Not bad for a fat boy," I thought to myself.

I got off the treadmill and was exhausted. I was sweating profusely. My legs felt as if they were tied to helium balloons, meaning I had to walk very slowly out of fear of falling over. I was very unsteady. Worst of all, I felt very light-headed. Had I overdone it? Probably, yes, but I didn't care because I had just run 10 kilometres.

Looking at myself in the mirror, which was not hard to do, since the gym was coated in nothing but mirrors from floor to ceiling, I could see that I was absolutely drained. I didn't look good, but I was still proud of my achievement.

This experience, taught me a very valuable lesson. I started thinking about *Ssh! Lifestyle20*. It was working so well and had got me to the point where I was fit and light enough to run for over an hour. I realised that if I continued to push myself in this way, even periodically, it would very likely start to form part of my routine.

Back to Basics

I knew then that this would not be sustainable. If I introduced an hour's run every month, or a 40 minute run every weekend, I knew that I would not keep it up, long term. It was a very important lesson. Push yourself, by all means, but come back to basics and say, "It's only 20 minutes every other day – that's all that is ever required."

If that 20 minutes becomes easy, because your fitness levels are higher and you are stronger, then that's great! Take advantage of that, but keep coming back to the all-important 20-minute rule. This is the key to sustainability. Now, when I feel like pushing myself, I remind myself of the essence and fundamentals of *Ssh! Lifestyle20*, which stops me from doing too much.

If we put this into practical terms and you do set yourself ambitious goals, like running a half-marathon or even a marathon, the likelihood is that you will exhaust your body and it will need time to recuperate.

After completing such an event, you will have to take time off to recover. It is easy to get into bad habits and taking a couple of weeks off Stage 2 of the Activity Plan can easily lead to three weeks off, then four and before you know it, you will be back to square one.

This is why Stage 1 (be more active) and Stage 2 (dedicated activity) work so well in conjunction with each other. If you want, or need, time off from Stage 2 (your 20 minute end-game), concentrate on Stage 1. Make sure you continue to be active in other areas of your life.

The whole point of *Ssh! Lifestyle20* is that it's exactly that: a lifestyle. It should be a habitual part of everyday living.

Active Planning

Planning is, again, a key aspect of fulfilling the Activity Plan. You do not want to allow yourself any excuses or the option to quit.

So, what arrangements have to be made to execute Stage 2 of the Activity Plan?

Here is what I did. These things might sound trivial, but, again, it is having the little things organised well that allows you to concentrate on the more challenging aspects of being active.

My planning consisted of the following:

- Buying a pair of trainers. When I first started out, and very much with "No excuses" in mind, I ran with what I had: a pair of what I would call fashionable trainers. They were totally inappropriate for running in, but, they got me out of the house.
- Getting a pair of headphones that would not be annoying when running, i.e. a large pair that would not easily fall off whilst jogging. I found that headphones that were placed in the ears kept falling out, which was very annoying.
- I had no suitable jogging clothes, so I needed to get shorts and t-shirts that were comfy to run in and not too heavy. As it was, I never did get

round to this and still have not done so. I run in a pair of swimming shorts! I do this because I did not want it to form an excuse. Running in swimming trunks is better than not running at all.

- Style – don't worry about it. You don't have to look good or stylish. Remember that it is not about what others think. *Ssh! Lifestyle20* is secret, so as long as you get out there and be active, that is all that matters.
- When someone sees you running, don't be concerned about what they might be thinking. I used to ponder about others' thoughts, but now have no time for that. They have no notion of the end-game and where you are on the path to achieving it. They will never see the finished article. If you are concerned that they might be laughing behind your back, let them. You will have the last laugh.
- If at all possible, do your jogging in a park, so that you have a nice setting – it helps, plus there are not usually many people around to spy on you.
- When you are jogging, remember to look around and enjoy your surroundings. I found that I concentrated so hard on the music and the physical process of running that I forgot to lift my head and take in what was around me. This helps.
- Get a supply of elastic bands and put them near the front door. That way, you can easily tie up the headphone lead to stop it from bumping about and annoying you while you run. I also tucked the excess lead into my shorts, which provided the same result.
- I use my iPhone for listening to music. Whatever device you use, get a holder for it, so it easily clips on to your clothing. I actually put it in the

pocket of my swimming shorts and I fold the pocket back on itself, so that the iPhone does not jump about too much. Alternatively, get yourself a small, light music device that won't move around when doing your active plan.

- As I have mentioned previously, time is precious to me, as I am sure it is for many people. Therefore, plan carefully when to fit your 20 minutes in. If you go out before work, you can kill two birds with one stone, because after you finish the run, you can shower, get ready for work and leave. Perfect. Because I go after work, when I get back from running, I quite often leave it until the next morning before I shower. Disgusting, maybe, but it does mean that the whole active routine, from start to finish, takes no longer than the 20 to 25 minutes. This is the all-important part for me. Consider all your options to make *Ssh! Lifestyle20* easy for you to sustain.

- Make sure that your total routine lasts no longer than 30 minutes. This includes getting ready, warming-up, running, showering and changing. I would say 30 minutes at the very most – ideally you should aim for 25 minutes. For longevity's sake, it would be better to have an end-game active plan of 15 minutes, so that the total time required is 20 minutes, if this means it will be sustainable for you.

- Running in the dark or at night is something that you are going to have to do, especially if you live in the UK and want to continue *Ssh! Lifestyle20* throughout the winter months. If you can, first run in the light, so that you can familiarise yourself with the route's hazards, such as potholes, curbs and uneven surfaces. This will minimise the possibility of sudden movements on the run and injury. Again, accept no excuses. If you have to run in the dark on your first time out, it is not a massive risk to take, so you should still go ahead, although I would recommend wearing light-coloured or reflective clothing if running on roads.

- If you feel unsure about running outside in the dark, run in your garden, or indoors on the spot, or up and down your stairs. Make the Activity Plan work for you. Again, no excuses.

- I found that during the colder nights, I wanted to run in a hooded top to keep warm. However, the hood kept falling off while I was jogging. The large headphones I use have a strap across the top of my head, so I stuck a piece of Velcro onto the top of that strap. I then sewed the other piece of Velcro into the top of the hood. Hey presto – my hood now stays up while I run. It's the little things that make this whole experience tolerable, so plan to allow you to succeed.

- You can use technology to help you with your activity plan. There are running apps that will tell you how fast and how far you are running. I use a free app called *Goal Getter*, but there are many on the market. The only caveat to this is that you must not rely on these gadgets. You need to keep it simple, so that you do not leave yourself open to excuses.

- If you have a partner and children, because the dedicated activity only requires a commitment every other day, you can alternate Stage 2 of your plans, which means, there is always someone to look after the kids. A great benefit of *Ssh! Lifestyle20*.

- You know what works for you. You might only want to commit to five minutes every other day. If you do less in Stage 2 make sure you commit to more in Stage 1. You know what's right and what is sustainable for you. You will know what makes the difference, so listen to yourself and no one else. Use the tools and personalise the Activity Plan.

Getting Cocky

It is important to warm-up your muscles before doing any energetic activities. This is simply common sense. I didn't really know what or how to warm-up my muscles when I started *Ssh! Lifestyle20*, but I now have a quick and clear routine that I go through before I leave the house.

When I began the last of my micro-goals (20-minute runs), I was not warming-up. 10 minutes into my first ever 20-minute run, I pulled my calf muscle. My body was not ready for the shift from 15 to 20 minutes, or I had tried to go too fast. Either way, I was getting cocky and eager to burn that fat away. Warming-up, I am positive, would have prevented this painful event.

Following this experience, I decided to formulate a fast and effective warm-up session.

Warm-Up

I stand on the balls of my feet on the bottom step of the staircase, so that most of my feet are hanging over the edge. I lean forward and put my hands on the stairs, a few steps up, so that I am stable. Then, I slowly tip my lower body backwards, so that I can feel the muscles in the back of my legs stretching.

I hold that for a count of five and I repeat another four times (five in total). If you would rather, or live in a bungalow, you can achieve the same results by standing on a book and holding the back of a chair for support. This warm-up works well for me and prevents muscle injury when I run.

Sometimes, I want to get the 20-minute routine over as quickly as possible, so I do not stretch my muscles before leaving the house. On these occasions I simply make sure that I go slowly for the first five minutes and this then acts as my warm-up. It means I do not go as far during the run, but more importantly, it prevents injury.

I can now tell whilst running when my body has warmed-up and when I can start running faster, without the danger of injuring myself.

Respect Injury

If you do get injured, you must respect that injury. When I pulled a muscle, it was hard for me, because I felt as if I was going to lose the battle and the war. I didn't want to have a week off, because I was worried I would not be motivated enough to start Stage 2 of the Activity Plan again.

There was nothing that I could do apart from rest. It took 10 days to recover completely. I wanted to get back to the running after seven days, but I also did not want to risk further injury. I made sure that the injury was 100 percent better before I started Stage 2 of the Activity Plan again.

It was during my recovery that I knew *Ssh! Lifestyle20* was working, because I actually missed not doing the 20-minute runs. This amazed me. It also got me thinking how important Stage 1 of the Activity Plan is. It is very important to supplement your dedicated 20-minute activity (Stage 2), and I will talk about this in more detail a little later on.

Any Niggles?

As an injury-prevention measure, I recommend that you monitor yourself while you run. What I mean by this is that when you are out running, concentrate on the muscles that you are using and monitor their performance. If you feel any signs of pain, any niggle at all, listen to your body and respect that it is trying to tell you something.

I did not listen. In hindsight, I did feel something before I pulled my calf muscle. If you do not actively monitor yourself and act on any slight complaint, it might lead to chronic injury. So, either slow down or stop completely.

With chronic injury, there are usually subtle telltale signs that make themselves known before the event occurs. You need to train yourself to recognise these.

If I feel that I might be on course for another injury, I will often stop early and walk home, or at least slow down and monitor the situation carefully. This way, I still complete my 20 minutes and get home without any further injuries.

If you do sustain an injury – and you might – you should also make this form part of your secret way of life. After my calf injury, my story was that I was playing football with my son in the garden. It will stop the questioning and leave you in a position of strength once again. Do not give too much away too early on.

Warm-Down?

People tell me that it is also important to warm-down after a workout. I have never done so. 20 minutes is the most physical exertion I ever do, so I have found that the muscles generally don't need to work off that amount of effort.

What I do quite often, as a form of warm-down, is to get into a hot bath, put my legs flat on the base of the bath and then lean forward to stretch the muscles in the backs of the legs. I will also get into a kneeling position and sit down on the backs on my legs, resting my weight, for about 10 seconds, to stretch the muscles the other way as well.

Relaxing in a bath and thinking about how I have just completed another little step on the path to a thinner and healthier body is the best type of warm-down I know.

I'm Hurting!

Sometimes, it really hurts. My muscles ache, my Achilles tendons hurt and, mentally, that makes it all the more difficult. Other times, you will find that you feel strong and the 20 minutes goes by very easily, because your body is not suffering, you feel positive and, dare I say it, you might even enjoy the time that you are out.

When you experience this positivity and your body does feel strong, use it to your advantage. I recommend that you run faster but not for longer. Stay true to your goal. Run for 20 minutes, but make sure that you cover a greater distance. This way, you can sustain Stage 2 of the Activity Plan and also work your body harder, which will mean that you become fitter, burn more calories and lose more weight.

On the flipside, the hardest times are when you feel weak and demotivated. My advice is to respect these feelings, be proactive and react to them. Listen to your body, as you do when monitoring yourself for injuries.

On these days, do not run as fast or as far. Still try to complete the time for the goal that you are on, but don't overdo it. Give in to your body.

If you are unwell, it is another time to listen to your body and rest. Rest is fine. During the times that you are not taking part in Stage 2, concentrate on Stage 1 and make sure that you are being more active in the other areas of your life. This simply makes *Ssh! Lifestyle20* more sustainable.

Where to Go?

As with other areas of *Ssh! Lifestyle20*, making the process a habit helps tremendously. I always run the same route, whilst listening to the same songs, every time I go out.

There are three reasons for this:

1. I know the distance that I am running.
2. I can gauge where I am in my run, or more accurately, how far until I reach home.
3. I run in a park near my home and I enjoy the surroundings.

If you want to know how far you are running, then there is the tried and tested way of getting in a car and driving the route to measure the distance on your speedometer.

However, these days, it is easy to go online. There are many websites that will calculate the distance of your route, such as www.mapmyrun.com and www.goodrunguide.co.uk. You can simply drag and drop a pointer onto a map or satellite image. If, like me, you run in parkland, you can easily mark out the route, and it will calculate the distance. The other way is to get an app for your phone which can work out the distance as you jog.

Supplementary Activities

You should also supplement the running with as much extra activity as you can. This gives added flexibility to *Ssh! Lifestyle20*, especially on the days that you might have to miss your dedicated activity. It also helps if you do injure yourself, because you will have other activities to call upon, to help you achieve the end-game.

To be very clear: do not rely on these supplementary activities. Once you have gained a certain level of fitness, you might want to partake in more enjoyable physical activities, such as football, badminton, hockey, tennis or rugby. However, do these as an extra. **Do not** let them be your only source of activity.

Team sports, by their very nature, require others to play with, and so others to rely on. One-on-one sports, such as tennis, badminton and squash, also require you to rely on others. If you want to play one-on-one games, do not let your partner's potential irregularity become an excuse for you.

You have to take responsibility. The 20-minute rule only applies to you. Do not make the excuse, "I cannot do it today because Harry let me down," or, for that matter, make any excuse. Keep the Activity Plan separate from any additional activities that you do.

Below are a few suggestions that can supplement your Activity Plan, and don't depend on others. Try to introduce one of these, or a selection, into your everyday life along with Stages 1 and 2. They are easy to add, because they don't take long to complete, so you can find a time to do them, without infringing on other enjoyable aspects of your life.

Sit-Ups

The same strength-building strategy applies, as in running. Start with one or two sit-ups and slowly build up over time. If you cannot do sit-ups, then do what I call 'sit-downs'. Start in a sitting position on the floor and slowly lean back, until you feel your stomach muscles working. Count to five slowly, and then release by either sitting back up or lying down on the floor.

Sit-ups are good because they provide definition and accentuate your weight loss. I started with groups of five and then quickly moved to 15 sit-ups per time. Within a couple of weeks, I was doing 30 at a time.

At a couple of seconds per sit-up, it shouldn't take more than a minute or two per day, so, make sure that you find the time to fit it into your schedule. Make it part of your routine when you are getting dressed in the mornings: underwear on, sit-ups, shirt on, clothes on and then downstairs for breakfast.

I do my sit-ups in front of a full-length mirror in the morning and I do my hair at the same time. I put the gel in and style it while I do the sit-ups. This works perfectly for me. Killing two birds with one stone ensures that the Activity Plan does not encroach on my life. It fits in with my lifestyle.

I am not going to do any more than 30 sit-ups, because it will consume too much of my time. If I do more, I know it will become unsustainable.

If I forget or do not do the sit-ups during the mornings, I do them at night when I clean my teeth and use mouthwash. Otherwise, I would stand there and do nothing, so why not do the sit-ups at the same time?

Walking

As already mentioned in Stage 1 of the Activity Plan, walking is an excellent and easy way to be more active. I now walk more often. Walking is a really effective way of burning calories and losing weight. It simply takes a little longer for the results to be seen when compared to more physically active exercises.

Walking is the perfect supplementary activity. I get off the train one stop early on the way to work and walk. I don't do it on the way home, because I want to get home as soon as possible and I'd rather get home earlier and in to work later.

I do not have any specific plans or routines when walking, I simply walk if I am in walking distance, rather than using any other form of transport. I always do this.

Twists

Keep your feet rooted to the floor. Twist your upper body to the left and then to the right. This uses the muscle groups around your waist and, over the long-term, will provide definition.

I find twists really useful and totally un-energetic, which, as far as I am concerned, is perfect. They can also be done anywhere. I usually do twists whilst I wait for the kettle to boil in the morning, or while watching the television. Simple!

Press-Ups

I do not do these, but they might work for you. As always, work up slowly and find a time and place where you can do them without disruption.

Kneeling, instead of resting your body weight on your feet, when doing the press-ups is a good way to build up the strength in your arms, without exerting yourself too much.

Star Jumps and Burpees

As above, I don't do them, but they might work for you. Ensure that you find a time to fit them seamlessly into your daily routine.

Equipment-Reliant Activities

By equipment-reliant activities, I mean sports such as, cycling and rowing. I don't take part in these, because they require additional planning, due to the equipment involved. Cycling can easily fit into your routine without too much extra planning, because it is an efficient way to get around. However, rowing requires a specific location, i.e. a lake or river!

If you are keen to introduce these types of activities, I suggest that you use the same methods that I do with walking. Fit them in as supplementary activities whenever you can, but do not allow them be your only source of exercise. What happens if you get a puncture, for example? It leaves you open to make a big excuse for not completing your plan. Common sense should prevail. Build these extras in to support your Activity Plan.

Anything you can do to supplement Stage 2 of the Activity Plan will help you achieve greater and faster weight loss. I found myself wanting to do more, which is positive, but I always come back to the central question: if I do more, can I keep it up over the long term?

You will soon start to notice your body change. It will take about six months for your body to adapt to the 20-minute routine and become strong enough so that it's not a struggle. Obviously, this will differ for everyone.

When you reach that level of fitness, getting out and being active for 20 minutes will become easier. If you still find it challenging, which you might, think of the fundamentals of *Ssh! Lifestyle20:* realise that it is your Time to Change and use the dominant themes of the Secret Lifestyle, Self-Evaluation, Planning, the Activity and Food Plans to help you achieve your end-game. I found it exhilarating to watch my body become stronger and more defined. You will also, I am sure, find the same.

Chapter IX

Step 7 – Weight Loss

*"Success consists of going from failure to
failure without loss of enthusiasm."*
Sir Winston Churchill

Stating the Obvious

To know if you are losing weight, you have to weigh
yourself. This is something that I have always hated
doing, partly because I am not interested or vain enough
to care and partly because the result has never been
quite what I was hoping for. However, it is important to
weigh yourself, especially early on, because it will drive
you forward.

When you realise that you are losing weight without
much effort, this will inspire you to continue with this
secret way of life. It will be the icing on the cake. You
will see with your own eyes that you are getting less and
less heavy.

It is the most exciting aspect of *Ssh! Lifestyle20.*

Importantly, it will also give you a method to monitor
and manage your micro-goals. If you are not losing as
much weight as you had hoped, then your Food and
Activity Plans may need to be adjusted.

So, what is your ideal weight?

Ssh! Lose Weight in 20 Minutes is a book from an
ordinary person's perspective. Therefore, I am going to
give you my view on how you will know when you have
reached your ideal, natural weight.

There are many charts and tools in the market that
allow you to assess your weight, many of which I am
very sceptical about.

BMI

BMI is not only an airline. It stands for Body Mass Index. BMI is defined as the individual's body weight divided by the square of his or her height. I have used BMI in the past and it defined me as obese. I used to think, "How can a generic measurement work for every individual? It takes none of my physical traits into consideration, apart from my height and weight." How can it be accurate? Surely, it is a dangerous practice to standardise everyone? At the very least, I thought age should also be considered.

The fact is, the BMI was accurate for me. I was obese and I now realise that I was simply in denial. I didn't want to believe the result. It was so much easier for me to deny the index's accuracy than actually do something constructive about reducing my weight.

BMI is a generic tool and therefore you should not use this alone in gauging if you are overweight. The England rugby team, based on BMI alone, would be classified as, clinically obese. They are super-fit, professional sportspeople. This, for me, justifies my scepticism of the index.

A very close friend of mine often jokes about me being not fat, but simply big-boned, and he has a point. There are some people who do have larger muscles because of their genetic makeup or, as a result of training, or both, like the England rugby team.

I recently went for a health check. As part of the check, the nurse measured my waist circumference. I questioned her about this (and my concerns of BMI) and she confirmed that the size of your belly is far more related to your health (risk of heart attacks, diabetes and cancer) than by BMI. This made total sense to me.

Eyesight

The best measurement tool is sight. Our waist size is something that all of us can make a judgement on, by simply looking. The people who call me Fat Al and Big Al, have not weighed me on a set of scales and measured how tall I am with a measuring tape. They simply noticed that I had a big belly.

It comes back to self-evaluation and how much you want to change your canvas. You know if you are overweight because when you step out of the shower and look at yourself, you are not likely to be happy with what you see. You try on a pair of trousers that 12 months earlier, fitted perfectly, only to find that they are now too tight. You don't like people making comments about your general looks, because you feel self-conscious about your weight. You see your belly overhanging the top of your jeans and that is the bit you want to change, not your BMI. You don't need a set of scales to reach this conclusion.

Body shape is just as important as BMI, and is something that BMI simply does not take into consideration. If you have well-developed muscles, you may find that you will fall into the category of obese, when in fact you may have a healthy body shape and very little fat. So, if you want to measure your BMI, use it with caution.

Natural Weight

I believe that every person has what I call a natural weight. I am convinced that natural weight is not just the physical weight that you are, it also encompasses your psychological mindset. You have to be mentally content with your weight or you will end up binging, snacking or, at the other end of the spectrum, not eating as you should. Therefore, you have to be happy with the weight that you want to be, otherwise you will not be able to sustain it. When I refer to natural weight, I don't just mean your physical weight, but also your current disposition.

Everyone's weight fluctuates daily, weekly and yearly. You will sometimes be heavier and other times lighter. It depends on a variety of reasons, which is why it is important to continually assess your weight. As long as you maintain your new plans and routines, your weight will continue to drop, until you reach your natural weight.

If you are overweight or even obese, as I was, then you will find that you quickly lose the excess weight that you are carrying. Your body will very quickly adjust to *Ssh! Lifestyle20* and you will soon reap the rewards.

You'll know when you have reached your natural weight because you will be content, like the way you look and notice that your weight has stop dropping. It will fluctuate minimally (within a few pounds) around the weight that you set as your end-game.

If your BMI still says that you are overweight, but you are content and like the way you are, after following *Ssh! Lifestyle20* and having lost weight, then you have reached your natural weight. As long as you continue with the Activity Plan, Food Plan and complete *Ssh! Lifestyle20*, you will be in a good place.

You, and only you, will know if you need, want, or can lose more weight. If you want to achieve a different end-game, then simply set the micro-goals that will allow you to achieve it. Remember: the end-game needs to be sustainable and your natural weight needs to be realistic.

After you've set your new micro-goals and got into the new routine, you need to stay true to them, otherwise you will find that your weight slowly rises back up. Every goal has to be achievable. If your end-game is unrealistic, you will not achieve it.

Psychological Advantages

One trick that will help is to always weigh yourself in pounds, not in kilograms or stone. The Americans have it right here. Pounds disappear much more quickly. There are 14 pounds in only one stone or approximately six kilograms.

It's a bit like travelling on the motorways on the continent. When you see 197 kilometres to Paris, it feels like a long way. However, after 20 minutes and 25 miles, the next signpost reads 157 kilometres to Paris. It feels as if you've come much further than you have compared with if you were travelling in the UK or the USA. Obviously, you have travelled exactly the same distance, but your perception is altered, so you feel as if you have travelled further.

If we put this into practice, when you lose half a stone, that is equivalent to three kilograms or, even more impressively, a whole seven pounds. That's a much higher number – wow! Congratulations!

I found this a big help when measuring my weight. If you measure your weight loss in large numbers, your confidence and your motivation will be much greater for your next goal.

I strongly recommend that you do this. Of course, it does involve some planning. You might have to buy yourself a set of digital scales that can display pounds, kilograms and stone. Please do not let this be an excuse. Any set of scales will do, but having digital scales might help you mentally manage your weight loss easier. I found that it did.

When I started *Ssh! Lifestyle20*, I really wanted to see weight loss immediately. I found that I was weighing myself every day and sometimes even twice a day. I really wanted to see the weight fall off, because I knew I was onto something that was working for me.

It soon became obvious to me that weighing myself should not be an everyday activity. To gain true insight into how much I was actually losing, I would need to weigh myself each week. And that is exactly what I did. Having said that, sometimes I do still jump on the scales midway between micro-goals, to see how I am getting on.

It is totally up to you to manage this. Looking back, I found that at the beginning, I needed the reassurance to see if *Ssh! Lifestyle20* was working (which it was). I wanted to monitor myself more closely and weighed myself every other day. This gave me the incentive to carry on and I got very excited about achieving the next goal.

In the early stages of *Ssh! Lifestyle20*, my end-game changed from 189 pounds (86 kilograms or 13.5 stone) to 175 pounds (79 kilograms or 12.5 stone), because I knew that I could achieve this, based on the regularity and speed at which I was already losing weight. I would not have known this if I had not been weighing myself on a regular basis.

At 175 pounds, I knew that I would feel much better both mentally and physically. It was my natural weight. This is why I changed my end-game goal.

What About Now?

I now only weight myself once per month. Once *Ssh! Lifestyle20* is entrenched, you will not want to, or need to, weigh yourself regularly. I recommend that you keep a track of your weight as a reference point, but more importantly, keep track of how your clothes are fitting, the number of notches you use on your belt, or the tightness of your bra strap. These are the critical measurements and, interestingly, the measurements that link more closely with the most contemporary measures around medical risk.

I don't need to stand on a set of scales so regularly now, as I did at the start of *Ssh! Lifestyle20*, to tell me if I am overweight.

Another thing that I found myself doing was looking at ingredients and nutritional information, on food packaging, a lot more than I used to, especially the Kcal count, and fat and sugar content. I now avoid doing this, because it is contrary to the theory of *Ssh! Lifestyle20*.

The point to *Ssh! Lifestyle20* is that you do not have to do the things that other diets deem mandatory. You do not need to count calories, E numbers or saturated fats. You just carry on with what you enjoy and count the steps to your end-game.

Ssh! Lifestyle20 is not about a completely new, yet unsustainable, regime. *Ssh! Lifestyle20* is about making tiny changes to what you do already. All *Ssh! Lifestyle20* asks is a small change to your daily food consumption and a commitment to being more active. If you start analysing every aspect of everything that you eat, this undermines a sustainable commitment to a change in your lifestyle.

Are You on a Diet?

At some point, it will be impossible to hide your weight loss from anyone close to you, or even from people who are not. In much the same way as when people find out about your Activity Plan, there is no point denying that you are losing weight.

Bear in mind that if and when you do tell people, they will judge you and keep tabs on you: "How is your diet going?" and, "Have you cut out carbohydrates? I tried that; it really works," or, "By the way, have you stopped dieting yet?"

When this happens, I say something along the lines of, "I am not on a diet. I have a lifestyle that works for me; have you thought about changing your lifestyle?" This puts the pressure back on them.

I always inform people that I am not on a diet, because *Ssh! Lifestyle20* is a lifestyle and fundamentally not a diet. This reduces the amount of inquisitive questions, as illustrated above, that people will have regarding your eating habits. It makes them even more fascinated about how I have achieved the weight loss and makes *Ssh! Lifestyle20* all the more enjoyable. I feel positive that you, will feel the same.

The Negatives

I should be honest and let you know that there are some negatives to *Ssh! Lifestyle20* and, in particular, to weight loss. I have to wear a suit to work each day and I own about 10 suits. Very quickly, I realised that the suits that I were wearing made me look comical – I looked like Charlie Chaplin. They were just too big. In fact, my whole wardrobe needed changing and suits are particularly expensive.

While this, in its own right, is very positive, it meant that I had to buy a whole new set of casual clothes and a couple of suits in smaller sizes. The good work that I was doing to my waistband was bad on my bank balance. I eased my displeasure at this because I was not paying a monthly subscription to any health club or weight loss scheme. My investment was in the shape of new clothes!

Brilliant!

When you do reach your personal, psychological and physical natural weight, you should congratulate yourself.

You have made it.

Ssh! Lifestyle20 has worked. Continue as you are and enjoy being fitter and healthier. Do not change anything else. *Ssh! Lifestyle20* has worked and is working for you. Well done.

Chapter X

Let the Weight Loss Begin

"Your goals, minus your doubts, equal your reality."
Ralph Marston

This book has given you an insight into how a very regular guy has lost weight. Following the steps within these pages, it is easy for anyone to do the same.

If I can do it, anyone can.

My perspective and explanation of how I have achieved weight loss will, I hope, help others at least start on a path to a fitter and healthier lifestyle.

You must want to change the way you look. However, this applies to whatever route you take to health and fitness. The difference with *Ssh! Lifestyle20* is that if you fail, it doesn't matter.

Ssh! Lifestyle20 allows you to fail, assess why you failed, then plan your new micro-goals to ensure that you succeed in reaching the end-game the next time you try. No one will know of the blip, the short-term failure. Re-evaluate your *Ssh! Lifestyle20*, set yourself a different micro-goal and start again the very next day.

If you find it hard to keep up every aspect of *Ssh! Lifestyle20*, then go back to basics. It is fine, for example, to simply concentrate on Stage 1 (be more active) of the Activity Plan. Introduce Stage 2 (dedicated activity), step by step, when you feel ready to do so. A more drastic measure would be to completely drop the Activity Plan and simply concentrate on the Food Plan, or visa versa.

However, it is important to remember that people who lose weight through diet alone force their bodies to go into survival mode, which actually causes the body to learn to conserve energy. Though they have decreased the size of the 'wood-pile' (food going in), they have correspondingly made the 'stove' smaller. If they then go back to their normal diet, the 'wood-pile' becomes proportionally larger than the stove and weight piles back on more quickly.

The best way for you to achieve and sustain weight loss is to commit to all aspects of *Ssh! Lifestyle20*, especially the Activity and Food Plans.

Longevity

Ssh! Lifestyle20 is a lifestyle change, so you need to create something that you can commit to long-term. It doesn't matter if you take longer to get to your end-game, especially if no one knows what your end-game is. No one but you can judge your progress.

If you want a short-term fix, then go on a diet.

You will have to be patient, especially if your goals are ambitious. You have to believe that this is a long-term lifestyle change. The end-game is for you and you alone. This is why you will be successful.

Ssh! Lifestyle20 is unique because it provides you with a toolset so that you can create your own manageable, sustainable weight loss plan, tailored for you, and you, alone.

The Circle of Life

This brings us back to where we started: *Ssh! Lose Weight in 20 Minutes* contains nothing but common sense and, because of this, 99 percent of what you have read, I am convinced that you will have agreed with.

What I hope to have achieved is to share the tricks and tips I used to create a sustainable, fitter and healthier lifestyle.

It is not difficult to do.

Many people that I talk to believe that losing weight is hard. They say, "Let me into your secret" and, "How have you managed to lose the weight? Please tell me."

It is not hard.

The challenges come when you want to sustain the weight loss. *Ssh! Lifestyle20* is sustainable because I am not asking you to do anything radically differently from what you already do every day. Anyone who truly wants to change the way they look will see 20 minutes every other day as a small sacrifice for the benefits it bestows.

I have been transparent about some of my experiences in this book; I do this because I want to encourage you to look at your own life and draw on your experiences to achieve the right frame of mind to build a new lifestyle.

I am convinced that losing weight is mostly psychological, which is why much of *Ssh! Lifestyle20* relies on planning, habit, routines and training yourself to think differently. Weight loss requires a shift in mindset. It is up to you to manage, so draw on your experiences to make *Ssh! Lifestyle20* a success for you.

There's no end to *Ssh! Lifestyle20* and you choose when to start. Think about your past and when you have tried to lose weight before. Is the concern that it didn't work previously why you don't want to start? Do you think that you don't need to lose any weight? Is that why you are not ready to start? Then why are you reading this book?

Are you denial? Look back at photos of yourself 10 years ago and see the changes. Really analyse yourself. Make sure that you look past the funny clothes and the different hairstyles; really **see** the extra weight that you carry today.

There is a proverb that summarises this point eloquently, "There are none so blind as those who will not see." Note the use of, *will not* meaning, 'does not wish to' or, 'refuses to.' Very pertinent.

Deny no longer.

Start right away. From your very next meal, leave a little food on your plate. Go out for a brisk five minute walk, today.

What is stopping you?

I hope this book gives you the foundation that you need to lose weight successfully.

Who Said That?

There is a reason for starting each chapter with a famous quote. I want to stress that anyone can lose weight with *Ssh! Lifestyle20*. I mean anyone. Someone very special in my life once said to me, "People will accept your ideas much more readily if you tell them that Benjamin Franklin said it first." I don't know the original author of this sentence but it doesn't matter, because it has stuck with me.

The challenges of weight loss remain the same for everyone. The challenges that present themselves when trying to lose weight are similar to other trials and tribulations of life. I wanted to highlight that these challenges and struggles are not unique. Many wise people have said many a wise word in support of others facing such difficulties.

I maintain that nothing in this book is unique. It is simply a different perspective or common sense, packaged in a way that has enabled me to face these challenges head on, and overcome them. Summarising each chapter with a famous person's viewpoint of the issues addressed reinforces the message that we all struggle from time to time.

It also gives the book some credence. People listen to the voice of authority. Because this is a normal person's perspective of an everyday challenge, starting each chapter with an authoritative quote emphasises the struggle. After all, people listen to Benjamin Franklin!

In Conclusion

Here are the six key messages from the book. They summarise what *Ssh! Lifestyle20* is and how I have managed to change my life by using them:

----

1. *Your body reflects who you are; it's your canvas. Be ready to change.*

2. *Keep Ssh! Lifestyle20 secret. This allows for multiple failures and enables us to reach the end-game goal. Treat each failure as a lesson.*

3. *Set micro-goals that are easily achievable. This way you will ensure that your path to the end-game is enjoyable and accessible.*

4. *Plan every minute detail and adopt a habitual lifestyle, so that you leave yourself with no excuses. Now, concentrate on the goal in hand.*

5. *Eat the same meals but eat less fat, carbohydrate and sugar. Don't be afraid to leave food.*

6. *Be more active – it's only 20 minutes!*

On the next page I also include a visual representation of the book, so that you can quickly remind yourself of how easy, it really is. If you only take onboard the actions on the chart you will succeed.

And remember, **the** most important key message is: it's only 20 minutes – that's all.

Can you really afford not to?

Ssh! Lifestyle20

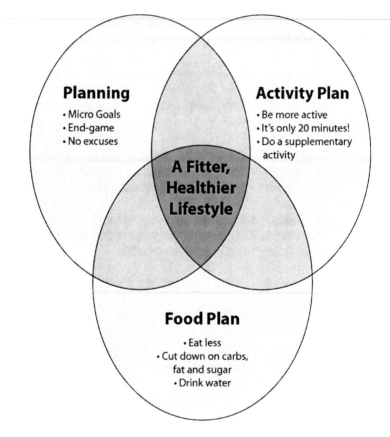

Enjoy your new lifestyle and keep it to yourself: *Ssh!*

References

'Who Moved My Cheese'
Spencer Johnson
Vermilion; New edition (7 Feb 2002)

'Winning!'
Clive Woodward
Hodder Paperbacks; Revised edition (6 Jun 2005)

The Food Standard Agency (FSA)
www.food.gov.uk

About the Author

Alex Buckley was born in 1970 in Crowborough, East Sussex. He now lives in Epsom, Surrey with his wife, Shauna and three boys, Jack, Oliver and Nathaniel.

Alex is a musician at heart. He started the trumpet at the age of 11 and went on to study music at Kingston University, where he obtained a 2:1 honours degree.

After university, Alex set-up Meteor Music, a music publishing firm, writing music for film and television. Clients included BBC, Channel 4, Channel 5, Rank Film Organisation and L!ve TV.

In 2000, Alex entered a televised competition hosted by Jon Snow called *The eMillionaire Show*. The prize was a £2m investment! Out of 7,000 applicants, Alex got through to the live final where he had to pitch his business idea to a panel of successful entrepreneurs.

Unfortunately, he did not win but following the programme he gained a substantial investment to start his business; com-poser.com. A year later the dot-bomb hit and com-poser.com required second round funding, something that was never going to happen in the, 'dotting like flies' climate.

This is when Alex turned to sales. He joined the company Venda, an eCommerce technology start-up and helped it grow into a world-leading eCommerce technology platform.

Alex has a passion for life and in particular food, which expressed itself in him becoming overweight. Alex formulated a plan that would enable him to lose weight which he found very easy to do.

Realising that he had stumbled on something that people were very interested in, he decided to write it down, in the hope that he could help others lose weight.

Follow Alex on Twitter: @SshLifestyle20
Website: www.sshbooks.com

Also from MX Publishing

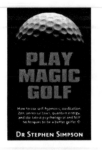

Play Magic Golf

How to use self-hypnosis, meditation, Zen, universal laws, quantum energy, and the latest psychological and NLP techniques to be a better golfer

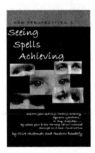

Seeing Spells Achieving

The UK's leading NLP book for learning difficulties, including dyslexia

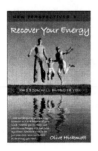

Recover Your Energy

NLP for Chronic Fatigue, ME and tiredness

More books at www.mxpublishing.co.uk

Also from MX Publishing

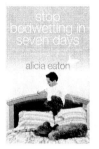

Stop Bedwetting in 7 Days

A simple step-by-step guide to help children conquer bedwetting problems in just a few days

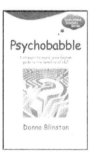

Psychobabble

A straight forward, plain English guide to the benefits of NLP

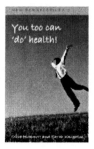

You Too Can Do Health

Improve your health and wellbeing, through the inspiration of one person's journey of self-development and self-awareness using NLP, energy and the secret law of attraction

More books at www.mxpublishing.co.uk

Also from MX Publishing

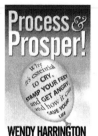

Process and Prosper

Inspiring and motivational book from necrotising faciitis survivor Wendy Harrington. Amazing book for anyone facing critical trauma.

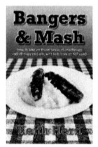

Bangers and Mash

Battling throat cancer with the help of an NLP coach. Keith's story has led to changes in procedure in many cancer hospitals and is an inspiration to cancer patients everywhere.

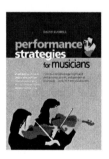

Performance Strategies for Musicians

Tackle stage fright and performance anxiety using NLP.

More books at www.mxpublishing.co.uk

Lightning Source UK Ltd.
Milton Keynes UK
177685UK00001B/2/P